THE SIRTFOOD DIET

*All About Sirtuins, the Skinny Gene,
and the Ultimate Healthy Recipes for
a Rapid Weight Loss*

Kate Longfield

owned by the owners themselves, not affiliated with this document.

TABLE OF CONTENTS

Introduction

The Sirtfood Diet is the latest trend in terms of diets, ever since Adele revealed her secret for rapid weight loss. After many other famous people claimed it to be helpful, the Sirtfood Diet became viral. We will see why.

Most people had to deal with diets at some point in their lives, for aesthetic or medical issues. There is a whole world of diets: Keto, alkaline, Mediterranean, and even hypnosis for weight loss. In my other book, I talked about the safety and the long-term results of the anti-inflammatory diet. It works!

Now it's time to see if the Sirtfood Diet also works. The most important aspect of this diet is that it doesn't deprive you of delicious food. It will be much easier to go along with it and enjoy your life. Let's put it this way: you will not feel guilty when you eat a dessert or when you finish your plate.

Because the results are great, you will feel encouraged and determined to follow your plan for losing weight. The Sirtfood Diet is all about enjoying your favorite foods, in the right quantities, of course. It is best to be combined with physical exercise, but not excessive ones. Jogging for half an hour is more than enough!

Each diet works, but it all depends on the person that is following it. The Sirtfood Diet is the newest arrival. We have plenty of testimonials that it works. Its creators claim that it activates the "skinny gene" in our bodies.

Besides making you lose weight, it will also help you live a happy, healthy life. It was created by British nutritionists Aiden Goggins and Glen Matten. They are the ones who started this sirtuins discovery. They focused on increasing the body's intake of sirtuins and calorie restriction.

It is all about sirtuins and foods that contain these proteins with high effects on metabolic regulation. It's all about genetics and how sirtuins help our body accelerate metabolism, improve digestion, and keep fit and energized.

Sirtfoods are those foods that contain high levels of sirtuins. It's not only fruits and vegetables- the favorite ingredients of most nutritionists. Think that you can eat chocolate, drink red wine, and enjoy the most exquisite recipes with fish, poultry, or pork. They are easy to find and affordable for everybody.

We will see that the most critical aspect of this diet is drinking a lot of green juice or tea. Drinking lots of fluids is another negative aspect- some nutritionists say. We will cover all these issues step-by-step!

The Sirtfood Diet is useful not only for weight loss, but also for its anti-aging properties, building muscles, cell regeneration, and keeping at bay some chronic diseases.

We will learn all there is to learn about sirtuins, the best Sirtfoods, the pros and cons of the Sirtfood Diet, the ways to maintain our weight, and how to shift our weight quickly without radical dieting. Some nutritionists claim that this is a radical diet, and that is easy to gain back the lost pounds once you finish it. We will get on that later!

We will learn about the best Sirtfoods, howto use polyphenols from our favorite foods, how to activate metabolism, and how not to deprive ourselves of vegetables, fruits, and favorite foods.

I will explain the two phases of the diet, and most importantly, how to maintain the weight. Consistency is the key!

Since it's about calorie restriction, it's advisable to get advice from your general practitioner or dietitian before starting your diet.

I also included a meal plan for 21 days, with the most famous and delicious recipes that anyone will love. You may even start cooking your dishes, which is great mental support for your struggle with a diet. It can offer you great satisfaction, therefore a happier lifestyle. Who is happy is also healthy!

We will get into the science beyond this diet, with studies and testimonials from people that followed this innovative diet. We will get to see if it is really sustainable and if it has long-term results or any side effects on our bodies.

Let's start our journey!

What are sirtuins?

Sirtuins are a group of seven proteins that protect the cells in our bodies from dying or becoming inflamed through illness, that help regulate our metabolism, increase muscle, and burn fat. They also regulate lifespan.

It's all about genetics. The main role of sirtuins is to select the key genes in our bodies and activate those responsible for metabolism, cell repair, defense, brain plasticity, and memory formation functions.

They orchestrate mechanisms deep inside our bodies that are essential mainly for weight loss and sensitivity to diseases.

So, the Sirtfood Diet is all about increasing the sirtuin-rich foods- certain natural plant compounds that can increase the levels of sirtuins in our bodies. Another trigger of high levels of sirtuins in our bodies is the calorie restriction. Therefore this diet works on the combination of these two factors.

Diet usually means restriction of food. Restriction leads to hunger, irritability, muscle loss, and metabolism slowdown. That's why the activation of sirtuins helps us achieve our goals in weight loss. No more starvation!

When sirtuins are activated, we make the most of caloric restriction and fasting. We are changing our cells' behavior, and that leads to increased metabolism, decreased inflammation, increased muscle efficiency, and damaged cells repair.

Sirtuins are found in every living organism on the planet and almost every part of the cells. They control what is going on by helping the cells react to external and internal changes.

The Silent Information Regulator 2(SIR2) is the formal name for this class of proteins. In humans, they range from 1 to 7 and are classified as class III histone deacetylases (HDAC).

According to this classification, SIRT1, SIRT2, and SIRT3 are part of class I, SIRT4 is class II,

SIRT5 represents class III, and SIRT 6 and SIRT7 belong to class IV.

According to their subcellular localization, we see that SIRT1, SIRT6, and SIRT7 work on the cell's nucleus, SIRT3, SIRT 4, and aSIRT5 in the cell's mitochondria, and SIRT2 works in the cell's cytoplasm.

Mitochondrial sirtuins are part of the sirtuin family of NAD+ dependant deacetylase and ADP ribosyl transferases. NAD+ is responsible for coupling the nutrient status of the cell with coordinated stress responses.

They also differ in function:

- SIRT1 is involved in glucose metabolism, neurodegeneration, aging, cell death, and tumorigenesis
- SIRT2 controls chromatin, DNA damage response, the gene expression regulation, and has the ability to deacetylase
- SIRT3 is responsible for ATP production, fatty acid oxidation, and mitochondrial protein regulation. It also controls caloric restriction and cellular response to oxidative stress.

- SIRT4 is involved in ADP-ribosylation
- SIRT5 has a desuccinylase activity
- SIRT6 is involved in the metabolism hemostasis, DNA repair, and genome stability
- SIRT7 regulates the transcription of the ribosomal genes.

Polyphenols

Polyphenols are the stress-response system of plants to extreme physiological stresses and threats over the past billion years. They had to produce a vast array of chemicals to adapt and survive.

In small words, when we consume plants, we absorb their polyphenols, which activate our innate stress-response system.

The polyphenols that we find in the Sirtfroods are micronutrients packed with antioxidants, and that helps our bodies improve digestion and neurodegenerative or cardiovascular diseases.

Sirtuins were first discovered through their effect on the fat cells. When the sirtuins turn on the short-term receptors that detect famine, the fat cells will start to metabolize and cause fat loss.

Studies have shown that when hunger strikes, the sirtuins repress the fat regulAtor genes controlled by PPAR-gamma.

PPAR-gamma(peroxide proliferator-activated receptor-gamma) is responsible for the fat gain mechanism by activating the genes required to start synthesizing food and storing fat.

The sirtuins come in to activate the "skinny genes". They stop developing and storing WAT(white adipose tissue). They use it for energy. In this way, the body's metabolism changes, so we get rid of excess fat. They also help fullness issues by making our body more sensitive to leptin- the satiety hormone.

How are sirtuins activated?

There are three ways to activate sirtuins in our body:

1. Histone modifications
As soon as you consume calories, the body goes into the survival mode. The cells are subjected

to a repair and maintenance program. Histones are proteins around which DNA is wrapped. Sirtuins start shutting genes down, by making sure that the DNA is no longer accessible. No gene is copied, and no gene product, such as enzymes, is produced.

This is how sirtuins influence the gene expression regulation and how the natural substances from our diet act on this very mechanism.

2. DNA methylation

DNA methylation is the attachment of methyl groups to nucleotides of DNA. The DNA represents the genetic fingerprint of an organism.

A gene can be deactivated by finding methylated nucleotides. That will ensure that no gene is copied. These enzymes that attach the methyl groups to the DNA are activated or disabled by sirtuins.

3. RNAs/ Non-coding (micro)

RNA is a super machine that regulates the activity of a cell.

WAT

The human body generally burns proteins and carbohydrates immediately, but stores specialized cells called white adipose tissue(WAT) for later use. When the caloric intake is reduced, the WAT stops storing fat and uses it for the metabolism.

That means that sirtuins help avoid fat from being stored in the body and prevent aging or other chronic diseases, such as diabetes, heart diseases, and even cancer.

WAT is responsible for the preservation of fat supplies, and it releases all sorts of inflammatory chemicals that prevent fat loss. It also promotes more accumulation of fat, keeping us overweight.

In this case, sirtuins activate BAT(brown adipose tissue) metabolism. BAT is thermogenic fat. We find it in small animals and babies, and it is a natural defense against cold temperatures. Animals use it to keep warm through rough winters. In humans, the considerable amounts contained in new-born babies will slowly decline with age.

Sirtuin stimulation will cause the BAT to be considered by the cells as WAT. The turned-on genes will see BAT as a new source of adipose tissue, and they will start to metabolize it. That will lead to fat being melted away. So, sirtuins help us expend energy and dissipate large amounts of fat.

The lean gene

There are no two people alike in the world. It is all about genetics. Our genes make us different! Not everybody has the "obesity gene", also called FTO.

Those who have this gene are prone to obesity, regardless of exercise or diet. The excuse of genetics is only an excuse for people to become lazy. They won't try to have a healthy lifestyle because they have it in their DNA!

Well, that is absolutely not true. You are predisposed to some disease, but if you do something about and stop creating bad habits, you could develop a healthy life gene. It only takes the will to build a healthy environment, so you don't come down with your genetics weakness.

Some research has found that people with the FTO gene are 70 % more likely to become obese. Why? Because they don't do anything about it!

Another interesting fact about our "obesity gene" is that sometimes an ideal weight is considered clinically obese, due to body fat. One can be skinny but has 30 % of body fat!

So maybe it's best to have our body fat composition tested. Body fat composition has a tremendous role in our diets. If we have a higher percentage of muscle mass, we can eat more. The key is to feed your body healthy foods! If you don't, your muscle mass will decrease so your body will not be burning fat so fast anymore.

The best ways to increase muscle mass are exercise and protein intake. This is where the Sirtfoods interfere with genetics. We can change our genes!

When we give our body the proper nutrition, our genes get turned on. In small words, the "obesity gene" becomes "skinny gene". This is the vital role of the Sirtfood Diet.

In the states, two of three people are overweight. Unfortunately, the numbers are getting higher each day. So the risk of diabetes, heart disorders, and other chronic diseases. We have to do something about it!

The solution is to search for inspiration from older societies that were healthier because of their eating habits.

The Asians and the Europeans are famous for their longevity and lean shape. They stick to good foods, daily exercise, and astress-free lifestyle.

How do sirtuins help us?

Outside Goggins and Matten's tests, scientific trials have shown promising results of sirtuin-rich foods. For example, researchers at Columbia University in New York found that drinking water with cocoa improved memory in middle-aged subjects.

Another study, in Melbourne, showed the effect of turmeric on the memory of subjects in the early stages of type 2 diabetes. It is all because sirtuin activation increases the amount of insulin that can be secreted.

Another asset of sirtuin activation in the body is the production and survival of osteoblasts.
The next best thing about Sirtfoods is their relationship with leucine, the primary muscle-builder amino acid. Goggins explains that "leucine is a double-edged sword because it is an accelerator for the muscle growth, but if you don't have the machinery to deal with it, the engine explodes."

When you come to think of it, it's mostly about eating well. If you put aside the calorie restriction of the first phase and jump to the maintenance one, you would be eating a wide variety of key foods in the world healthiest areas, such as Japan and Italy, where people live longer and have healthier lives.

So, we don't deal with superfoods, but with healthy natural ingredients.

Weight loss

Sirtuins are proteins that help our bodies burn fat fast. The creators of the Sirtfood Diet proved that you could lose 7 pounds in seven days. The hypothalamus is the central weight and energy balance controller. Therefore, the hypothalamic SIRT1 helps us lose weight because it modulates energy intake and energy consumption.

Another vital aspect of sirtuins is that they also increase the thyroid hormones release. That will lead to a better and faster metabolism.

One may think that it's best to use medicines that contain sirtuins, so the body is fooled into releasing fat without the side effects that come from radical dieting.

Most people turn to Resveratrol or Acai supplements, but their efficacy is doubtful. No study has shown that they promote weight loss or have any positive health effects.

Building muscles

Besides caloric restriction, exercise also helps sirtuin activation.

The sirtuins are responsible for burning fat rather than muscle for energy. They also improve the skeletal muscles (the muscles that one moves voluntarily), such as shoulders, back, limbs, and so on.

The skeletal muscles are usually used for any activity. The sirtuin-rich foods help us lose weight, but don't alter the muscle mass as fasting does. They actually help our muscles grow and find the energy to go along through sustained activity.

By activating sirtuins, we stop the loss of muscle mass and function. We will get to see multiple related health benefits, such as improved mobility, decreased inflammation, and bone deterioration due to aging.

It's not only for the elderly since signs of muscle aging start to show at the age of twenty-five. Slowly the muscle erodes, but sirtuins will help our bodies inhibit and reverse muscle deterioration.

Muscle regeneration is also the target of sirtuins. They are muscle regulators, so it will help our muscles grow stronger, stay healthier, and function better.

Appetite control

Another property of the sirtuins is releasing hormones like leptin, which controls the feeling of satiety. This is another asset for those who want to lose weight fast, in the safest way possible with this method.

The amount of leptin in the blood is important for appetite control. Sirtuins have the leading role in controlling how much leptin enters the brain, so it affects the hypothalamus in the right way. Increased leptin delivery to the brain causes overcoming leptin resistance. The hypothalamus will get the right signals from our taste centers and will respond with better control of appetite.

In small words, we will get more pleasure and satisfaction from our meals. This will keep us safe from overeating. We will no longer need extra food to be happy. That's why the Sirtfood Diet will never make you feel hungry!

Prevent diabetes

The activation of sirtuins also increases insulin production. That is helpful for our bodies since insulin resistance has a vital role in weight gain. When our body fails to react adequately to insulin, we only gain more weight.

Sirtuins make cells insulin sensitive. Therefore they will remove more glucose from the bloodstream.

Slow down the aging process

With age, the cells lose their ability to repair or heal. Sirtuins will help a cell quickly repair, improve, or reproduce itself. You will look not only younger but also feel young inside. By turning on and off specific genes, the sirtuins repair DNA damage. That leads to addressing particular sites of injury. As organisms age, the risk of DNA damage increases, so sirtuins focus on those areas.

There is the risk of creating gene confusion, so high activity of sirtuins may cause the body to "forget" what cells are to repair, and that only leads to further damage.

This is the reason that specialists try to make more studies, in a way to find the right levels of sirtuins in the body.

Increasing the consumption of sirtuin-rich foods could slow the aging process. Geriatrics are determined to study this aspect further. They are interested in chemical compounds- the right level of sirtuins in our bodies, and other biological processes. There is no question that

sirtuins help to slow down the aging process, reducing heart diseases, diabetes, and other age-related diseases.
We must also mention their role in reducing wrinkles.

Resveratrol, which we find in high levels in Sirtfoods, is the primary activator of the sirtuin gene. It will increase the deacetylation rate that controls whether a gene is turned on or not. In small words, it controls longevity.

 It is also a powerful antioxidant that removes free radicals, which are responsible for aging.

Sleeping better

Activating sirtuins will help our circadian rhythm, and that will ensure a night of better sleep.

Memory improvement

Some sirtuin-rich foods are known to be a great help to improve our short-term memory or to prevent cognition problems.

Prevent cancer

Some sirtuins act more like proto-oncogenes. They are tumor suppressors, but not in all cases. It depends on the type of cancer and the molecular context.

Maintain your skin fresh

Your face does not develop wrinkles too soon due to the antioxidant properties of sirtuin-rich foods.

What is resveratrol?

I already mentioned resveratrol and its effect on longevity. Let's go further to learn all we need to know about it.

We know it's a sirtuin activator and a powerful antioxidant. Antioxidants play an essential role in getting rid of free radicals. These are produced during the metabolism process and are mainly responsible for cell death.

It was discovered in the 1970s, and it solved the French paradox. Why do°F. rench people eat so many fatty foods in a more significant proportion than the Americans yet reported fewer heart disease incidents? This was a great question.

Well, the key is the mechanism by which it functions to reduce fatty acids. All thanks to sirtuin-rich foods, such as red wine. Red wine has lots of chemicals that help our body get rid of the excess fatty acids.

In red grapes, it can be isolated from the fruit's skin, seeds, and pulp. It is merely a chemical that arises in the plant to fight off the fungal and bacterial colonies.

It has been isolated in more than 70 other plant species, and it works through sirtuins, the chemicals responsible for gene activation. Once resveratrol acts on sirtuins, sirtuins will affect the anti-aging genes.

Resveratrol has been used to control heart diseases, some cancers, and mainly for overall health.

Researchers, Cabo and Sinclair, showed that resveratrol improved longevity in overweight and aged mice. Both studies, one in 2006 and the other in 2008, showed that resveratrol prevented obesity and age-related cardiovascular decline. It also has positive effects on motor coordination, better bone thickness, density, and mineral content. So, life was actually prolonged.

Some people already think of resveratrol as a fountain of eternal youth. No studies on humans have supported this theory, though! At least, not yet!

Everybody talks about the caloric restriction as to the key to dieting and weight loss. Not only do you lose weight, but also improve your heart's and other organs' health. Due to the way resveratrol works to implement our health while losing weight, it makes it as efficient as caloric restriction.

So, we talk about lowering our cholesterol, fasting glucose levels for people with diabetes, improving blood pressure, and reducing the fat stores in our body.

The scientist David Sinclair showed that activating the SIR2 gene, the gene responsible for controlling the DNA health, also helps us live a longer, healthier life.

Human studies have begun because all the pharmaceutical companies are excited about having chemical resveratrol on the market.

There are already a few, at a reasonable price, but for now, let's stick to natural sirtuin-rich foods.

The bottom of the line is that it is encoded in every human's genes to seek a way to live longer. We can do that with a quick and efficient solution- resveratrol, the scientists say!

Why? Because it helps us find the perfect health balance, it sustains all the necessary energy and makes us look better even at an old age.

So, you can eat all sorts of foods, in reasonable amounts, without depriving yourself or bearing side effects of starvation. A glass of red wine, a bar of chocolate, and some natural vegetables or fruits rich in sirtuins will do the magic for you!

Is the Sirtfood Diet sustainable?

Let's admit that a diet that lets you eat chocolate and drink wine is appealing to everybody. We have seen that it works (not for everybody) and why it works.

Some nutritionists are still skeptical, with all the testimonials from famous people- like Adele, Tom Brady, Mariah Carey, and others; who used it and lost weight. Why? They consider it a radical diet due to the calorie restriction and complain about a lack of research in humans.

Adele has reportedly tried the Sirtfood Diet, in 2017. She said it requires eating lots of Sirtfoods to regulate the body's metabolism, inflammation level, and aging.

The calorie-restrictive nature of the diet leads to no long-term weight loss results. She also said that cutting out alcohol and cigarettes, and performing Pilates exercises were a tremendous help for her current figure.

Football star Tom Brady drinks gallons of water daily and keeps away from eggplants or tomatoes.

Mariah Carey said she eats nothing but Norwegian salmon and capers every day. The lack of critical nutrients we find in foods like vegetables, fruits, and grains is bound to lead to no sustainable results.

Cleansing diets with only juices, fasting, or only one meal a day will never ensure our body the energy it needs to sustain our activities. Other stars like Christina Aguillera, Kim Kardashian, Beyonce, and many others claim to use calorie-restrictive diets, but nutritionists say there is no real science behind them.

They say that the Sirtfood Diet has its pros and cons. What diet doesn't? In the chapters ahead, we have seen the advantages. Now let's talk about the cons!

Erin Morse, a chief clinical dietitian, showed that sirtuins change metabolism, help with longevity and aging, in animals. Unfortunately, there are no human studies to prove the benefits of eating sirtuin-rich foods. She also says that research on this topic is emerging.

Marion Nestle, professor of nutrition, is also skeptical about the benefits of sirtuins. He says that sirtuins are proteins, so they cannot survive the stomach acid and digesting enzymes in the small intestines.

Other nutritionists are concerned about this diet's short time (it takes only three weeks to go through it).

The calorie restriction leads to muscle loss, and that leads to a slow metabolism rate, and that will make weight maintenance more complicated, a doctor says. Indeed, there will be no long-term results, she also claims. Once you finish the diet, all pounds you lost so far will be gained back.

The weight loss due to calorie restriction happens without a doubt, because when the body is deprived by energy, it uses the energy stores, more exactly glycogen. Glycogen needs water to be stored, so the use of energy stores means the use of water as well. So, we actually lose "water weight". As soon as the diet ends, the glycogen is stored again, so the weight comes right back.

This is how she explains the non-lasting effects of this diet. What is worse, she says, is that the body also lowers its metabolic rate, and that will cause your body to need fewer calories for energy.

Rick Hay, a nutritionist, also claims it is very restrictive. Because you have to cut out major food groups, your body will lack essential nutrients such as iron and calcium.

He also says that you would experience headaches, nausea, fatigue, and dizziness. He doesn't recommend it to those who had a complicated relationship with eating in the past.

All these specialists give us a bit of hope by admitting that more human studies are required to see the actual efficiency of Sirtfoods. From the way it looks, it undoubtedly aroused interest, so hopefully, soon, we will see if there is really any science behind the Sirtfood Diet.

What are Sirtfoods?

Sirtfoods are sirtuin-activating foods. They are all accessible in any corner of the world. These foods have enormous health benefits since they increase longevity and ensure a high-quality life.

On a diet, the central aspect is cutting calories. That comes at a cost! Each one of us knows that you are not feeling your best. In the long-term, exhaustion, irritability, and lack of rapid results will cause you to fail.

The Sirtfood Diet aims weight loss without long-term restriction in calories. We obtain that by eating Sirtfoods- foods rich in particular nutrients that will help our body use emergency energy stores, in addition to burning fat.

Sirtfoods were dubbed for the first time, in 2003, when some researchers found resveratrol in red grapes and wine. Its healthful properties made them study further.

Anyway, this is how it all started. We already know about the Mediterranean diet. Red wine is a must-have at each course of the day. Italians use it since ancient times.

Except for wine, other fruits and vegetables are used daily. Maybe that's what makes the Mediterranean lifestyle the best there is!

Let's get to our top Sirtfoods:

• **Kale**

Kale is rich in carotenoids, such as beta-carotene, lutein, and zeaxanthin. It is also a great source of vitamins, such as folate, magnesium, vitamin K, and vitamins C.

These nutrients are beneficial for eye health and immunity.

• **Red wine**

Considered the initial Sirtfood, red wine is an ancient remedy for heart diseases, common colds, and some chronic diseases.

The red wine is probably the most loved ingredient of this diet.

• Strawberries

Strawberries are very nutritious, are rich in fisetin- a powerful sirtuin activator, and help us decrease the risk of Alzheimer's syndrome, diabetes, osteoporosis, and heart diseases. They are also helpful in reducing the body's demand for insulin by turning the food into sustained energy.

• Onions

Onions are used for centuries for their anti-inflammatory properties. They help us regulate blood sugar. They have the highest polyphenol content, are high in vitamin B6, folate, and potassium, and are best used in their raw state.

• Soy

Soy has a long history in Asian diets. It is high in polyphenols and helping us keep at bay certain cancers, heart diseases, and bone loss. It is a great sirtuin activator.

• **Parsley**

It's one of the most popular herbs in the world. It contains zero fat and cholesterol but is rich in vitamins, minerals, dietary fiber, and antioxidants. It is also a source of vitamin K that promotes autotrophic
activity in the bones.

• **Extra virgin olive oil**
Olives are another ingredient of the Mediterranean diet. They help us eliminate the excess cholesterol in the blood, control blood pressure, are rich in dietary fibers, and provide essential vitamins and amino acids.

They are rich in potassium, iron, magnesium, phosphorus, and are very nutritious.

• **Dark chocolate (85% cocoa)**

To stay healthy, you should eat dark chocolate. It has health benefits, such as decreasing the risk of heart disease and high blood pressure. It is high in fat and sugar content, so limit yourself to three bars a week.

• Green tea

Green tea contains potassium, vitamins, folate, caffeine, and other antioxidants. It helps us lose weight, reduce cholesterol, combat cardiovascular disease, and prevent Alzheimer's syndrome.

• Buckwheat

Buckwheat is one of the most popular crops in the entire world. It is high in proteins, manganese, potassium, zinc, rutin, and it is naturally gluten-free.

• Turmeric

It has anti-inflammatory effects and is a powerful antioxidant. It is used for a large area of digestive disorders, liver problems, kidney problems, and even depression.

• Walnuts

Walnuts are also the oldest tree-food. They are high in calories, vitamins such as magnesium, zinc, manganese, calcium, iron, and fats. They are a powerful sirtuin activator and help us reduce weight and the risk of diabetes or heart diseases. They also help the brain because they can reduce the risk of degenerative diseases and slow brain aging.

• Arugula/Rocket

Arugula, also known as rocket, is a top ingredient of the Mediterranean diet. It is high in vitamins, has digestive and diuretic properties, and contains quercetin and kaempferol, which help promote collagen synthesis in the skin.

• Omega-3 fish oil

Omega-3 fatty acids present in tuna, salmon, bluefish, sardines, and sturgeon have great health benefits.

• Garlic

Garlic, just like onions, is an ancient food used for its healing properties. It is a natural antibiotic used for rejuvenating powers, enhancing immunity, and treat stomach ulcers.

It helps lower the blood pressure level and for well-being in general.

• Medjool dates

Medjool dates are simply a natural source of sugar and polyphenols.

• Red Endive

Endives are the best addition to your salad. They have a bittersweet taste but are rich in luteolin- a great sirtuin activator. It has properties the help our brain remain healthy. Some specialists started using it to improve sociability in autistic children.

• Blueberries

Blueberries are rich in antioxidants and help reduce the risk of heart failure, strokes, and diabetes.

• Capers

Capers are high in rutoside and quercetin, strengthening capillaries and inhibiting clump formation in the blood vessels. They are a consistent source of vitamins.

• **Coffee**

Coffee is an excellent sirtuin activator, rich in nutrients and polyphenols. It helps decrease the risk of diabetes, certain cancers, and neurodegenerative diseases. It also protects the liver and has an important role in the fluid intake of the body.

The Sirtfood Diet

These are the tested Sirtfoods so far. We have seen the health properties they have. Think of combining them into a whole diet!

We have seen that Asian and Mediterranean lifestyles are the greatest. These natural diets, with all those leafy greens, spices, fruits, and red wines, are a valid help in maintaining a lean body; and a healthy heart and reducing the risk of obesity and diabetes.

Since not all vegetables and fruits are equally created, researchers came up with the idea to make all sorts of combinations.
What lacks to a vegetable, a fruit adds. In this way, sirtuin activation is ensured. That leads to increasing the benefits of each ingredient. Long-term benefits too!

A healthy lifestyle= weight management =disease reduction.

So, the Sirtfood Diet is a potent tool for those who are sick and tired of depraving themselves of all joys of life!

The pilot study conducted by the two creators of this innovative diet had great results. In only seven days, 39 participants of 40 lost an average of 7 pounds and gained or simply maintained the muscle mass.

The calorie restriction is the central part, but daily exercise contributed also.

The skeptics claim it is a radical diet and that the short time will never ensure the long-term effects on our body. Only a week indeed seems ridiculous!

In fact, the two dietitians have a program that takes three weeks (phase 1, phase 2, and maintenance). They actually advise you to keep up with this lifestyle and not give it up as soon as you find that you lost the pounds you wanted to.

The real purpose of this diet is to pack one's meals with as many sirtuin activators as possible. If you don't get a hold on the main ingredients at least, try to "sirtify" your meals, adding or substituting natural ingredients with Sirtfoods.

How does the Sirtfood Diet work?

There are two main phases: phase 1- it takes seven days, and phase 2- the most important, maintenance. It will take an extra two weeks.
The best start for the Sirtfood Diet is the green juice. So, I came up with this recipe. The two creators of the diet recommend drinking three juices and adding one meal for the first three days, then two meals and two juices for the next four days.

The Sirtfood green juice

- 2 large handfuls of kale
- a large handful of arugula
- a small handful of parsley leaves
- 2-3 large stalks of green celery
- 1/2 medium green apple
- the juice of 1/2 lemon
- 1 tsp of green tea

All you need to get started are those ingredients and a juicer. Start with kale, arugula, parsley. If you find that the green leaves are not correctly juiced, just go through the process again. The purpose is to obtain 50 ml of juice from our ingredients.

The next step is adding the celery, ginger, and apple, to reach about 250 ml. Now, you can peel the lemon and add it in the juicer or simply squeeze it by hand into the juice.

When the juice is ready, you should add the green tea and stir it with a teaspoon.

Once the matcha is dissolved, add the remainder of the juice. With a final stir, your green juice is ready to drink. If you wish, feel free to top up with water.
Serve and enjoy!
It is recommended to take the juices at different times of the day, and then have a meal for lunch or dinner.

It's best to use green tea only in the first two drinks of the day because it contains caffeine. Also, you are free to add water to it if you like.

Phase 1

For the first three days, one should consume three juices and one full meal, for a total of 1000 calories a day. From the forth day to seventh, you should increase your calories uptake to 1500 by consuming two green juices and two meals a day.

It is easy to follow other green juices recipes. Feel free to try vegetarian or vegan recipes.

The choice is yours!

Phase 2

Phase 2 includes other extra two weeks of Sirtfoods intake. Maybe no one told you, but by now you realized that Sirtfoods are for life. It is not a harmful method, but consistency is the key to get long-term results. Why not? We eat foods we like, get the most of our favorite greens, and obtain spectacular weight loss results.

Mindset is important! We do not starve ourselves! We do not deprive ourselves of the foods we like! Our bodies don't need all these calories to go ahead! It is only about following a diet that helps us burn fat fast and maintain a healthy lifestyle.

Phase 2 is actually about maintaining the fat loss results and keep on losing weight gradually. When you look at yourself in the mirror, you will see a better self, a leaner shape, and a toned body. That will give you the right input to go along.

You must realize that the 14 days maintenance plan will help you lay the foundations for a healthy future lifestyle.

The amazing thing about the Sirtfood Diet is that you not only lose weight, but you also build muscle. As I mentioned before, we don't have to fall into the scale trap. We don't have to weigh each day. This goes for all diets, especially for this one because the weight you lose is the one you don't see on a scale, but in the mirror.

Your body has already changed shape, it has toned up, and if the scale shows you the same numbers in the second week, it's because of the increased muscle mass.

In this phase, you will consume three meals, one green juice, and two optional Sirtfood snacks a day.

There are no time rules, but it's best to have your dinner by 7 PM.

During this phase, you will come to realize that portions are no longer an issue. You will feel well-fed and well-nourished. That's why it is essential to listen to your body. If you are already full before you finish a meal, then stop eating!

As for drinks, besides green juices, you can always add water, coffee, or tea. Let's not forget about the red wine, the top of the Sirtfoods. But keep in mind to use it in small amounts. For the beginning, for example, you should consume one glass of red wine for two to three days a week.

The good thing about phase 2 is that we return to the classic three meals a day. We all know that a good breakfast gives us energy and helps us stay focused. It also helps our bodies keep the blood sugar and fat rates in control, all due to metabolism.

Who eats late in the evening doesn't allow his body the time it needs to synthesize foods, so belly fat is back on track!

The snacks are another good thing about this diet. With three meals a day, one should be more than satisfied, but sometimes the brain sends the wrong signals when stressed, and we tend to find food safely. In these particular moments, a snack is a solution.

The treats are made entirely from Sirtfoods: dates, turmeric, walnuts, and extra virgin olive oil.

It is best to use no more than two a day, and only when it is necessary.

Other Sirtfoods

We have already seen the benefits of the top Sirtfoods. Now we will try to see how other foods can supplement our meals. By now, you already lost weight, you already learned how to use Sirtfoods for your goal, and the only thing you need right now is variety.

It's about maintaining your healthy lifestyle and add a bit of spice to your life!

So, let's talk about variety. The berries group includes not only strawberries and blueberries, but also black currants, raspberries, and blackberries. All these have significant amounts of sirtuin activator proteins.

As for the walnuts, we can also use chestnuts, pistachios, peanuts, and pecans.
When we talk of grains, not everybody agrees that they are healthy. Studies have shown that they are related to decreased inflammation, heart disease, diabetes, and even cancer. Of course, it's for the best not to eat the refined grains, but the whole grains, if possible.

I came up with a list of other foods that can help you maintain your weight, continue slowly losing weight, and vary your meals.

Vegetables:

- broccoli
- green beans
- watercress
- asparagus
- white onions
- yellow endive
- artichokes

Nuts and seeds:

- sunflower seeds
- chia seeds
- chestnuts
- pecan nuts
- pistachio

Fruits:

- apples
- cranberries
- black plums

- red grapes
- raspberries

Beans:

- fava beans
- white beans

Grains:

- quinoa
- popcorn
- whole-wheat grains

Herbs and spices:

- cinnamon
- oregano
- sage
- ginger
- peppermint
- thyme
- chives

You will see in the 21 days meal plan how these new foods can be "sirtified". It only means cooking something you like the most and using the right spice or dressing that will help your body activate sirtuins, to get the most of your favorite foods. This way, you will never feel deprived, and so the diet will be much easier to follow.

Animal-based proteins

We talked about vegetables and fruits. Now, let's talk about meat, eggs, fish, and dairy products. For those who are not vegetarian or vegan, these proteins give additional support for the body, and most importantly, they give you the satisfaction of not giving up on your favorite steak!

With these foods, we add proteins, such as leucine, mainly found in pork, red meat, eggs, and dairy products. They become extra help for our body to defeat obesity, diabetes, and certain cancers.

The important thing is, though, to keep away as much as possible from processed meats.

Animal-based proteins that come from dairy products are quite essential for the body since they are highly nutrient.

Milk may be a problem for those who suffer from lactose intolerance. Many people have this problem, but they already know about it, so it's safe to keep it away if that is the case. If no, drinking a glass of milk or adding a bit of sour cream, Parmesan, or Cheddar cheese for dressing your salads is the right kick to your ordinary diet.

The poultry, turkey, and fish are OK. As for the red meat, not everybody agrees to be that healthy. Anyway, if properly cooked, for example, marinated with herbs and then grilled or fried with a bunch of onions and olive oil should be more than enough to keep us away from the risk of certain cancers. The important thing is always not to overindulge on it.

Eggs are high in cholesterol, but at the same time, are an essential source of proteins. The cholesterol, as you know, is a trigger for heart diseases. That's why all specialists advise us to restrict the use of eggs. Don't worry, eating one, maximum of two eggs a week is no source of diseases.

Fish works for vegetarians also. For pescetarians, it is the only abundant source of omega-3 fatty acids. They have effects on heart diseases and have anti-inflammatory properties. They are also known as brain food- already used as a treatment for dementia and brain repair. Omega-3 fatty acids help stabilize the heart's electrical activity and lower blood pressure.

That should be all about Sirtfoods. Let's see how to combine them in the best way possible, so we have a most varied meal plan for at least 21 days!

Feel free to change or to add anything that comes in mind. Variety is essential!

A three-week meal plan

So, we have seen how Sirtfoods help us lose weight. Let's see how to plan a sustainable diet.

The first week

The first week is the harder one. Until you get used to the new foods to eat and get the right mindset to follow your diet, it may become bumpy. Keep your focus, and remember, you must achieve your goals!

Day 1
- Three green juices
- One main course:
    - Chicken salad
    - Fried shrimps with buckwheat noodles

Day 2
- Three green juices
- One main course:
    - Kale and red onion with buckwheat
    - Chicken breast with kale, red onion, and red salsa

Day 3
- Three green juices
- One main course:
    - Tuscan bean stew
    - Miso-marinated baked cod with stir-fried greens and sesame

Day 4
- Two green juices
-Two main courses:
    - Sirt Muesli
    - Sesame chicken salad
    - Grilled beef with red wine, onion rings, garlic, kale, and herb-roasted potatoes

Day 5
- Two green juices
- Two main courses:
    - Sirt salmon omelet
    - Sirt super salad
    - Chicken skewers with satay sauce

Day 6
- Two green juices
- Two main courses:
    - Strawberry buckwheat
    - Lentil Sirt super salad

- Chicken, kale, and sprout stir-fried

Day 7
-Two green juices
- Two main courses:
- Mushroom scrambled eggs
- Chicken, broccoli, and beetroot salad with avocado pesto
- Buckwheat noodles in a miso broth with tofu, celery, and kale

I forgot to mention the extra bar of dark chocolate(no more than four a week) you can add to your main course and the glass of red wine that will undoubtedly soothe you in the evening!

The second week

The second week of our diet is a bit easier. We return to three main courses and only one green juice a day. Now we talk about breakfast, lunch, dinner, and snacks.

Breakfast

Now we have more choices, besides the green juice. Breakfast should be the essential course of the day, so let's start with something outstanding!

We can choose from:

- Sirt muesli

- Yogurt with mixed berries, chopped walnuts, and dark chocolate

- Spiced scrambled eggs

- Buckwheat pancakes with strawberries, chopped walnuts, and chocolate sauce

- Coconut yogurt with mixed berries and chopped walnuts

- Sirtfood omelet

-Apple pancake with blackcurrant compote

- Fruit salad

- Smoked salmon omelet
- Kale and blackcurrant smoothie

- Date and walnut porridge

- Kale omelette
- Fruit smoothie with rolled oats and soy milk

Lunch

Here you can vary all you want. I will give you some ideas. The choice is yours!

- Tuna sirt salad

- Chicken sirt salad

- Strawberry buckwheat tabbouleh

- Waldorf salad

- Buckwheat pasta salad

- Chicken and soba noodles stir fry

- Sirtfood pizza

- Lentil sirt salad

- Tofu and shitake mushroom soup

- Red endive, pear, and hazelnut salad

- Prawn arrabiatta

- Italian kale

- Turmeric baked salmon
- Kale salad with edamame beans and red onions dressed in olive oil

- Sirt beef burgers

- Butternut squash, and date tagine

-Rocket salad with tuna, tomatoes, and cucumber dressed in olive oil

- Spicy chicken curry with wholegrain brown rice

- Grilled fish with buckwheat salad

Dinner

For dinner, the best choices are soups, but fish plates do their job too. They are light courses. The body takes less time to synthesize the nutrients.

You can choose from:

- Greek salad skewers

- Fruit salad

- Asian shrimps stir-fried with buckwheat noodles

- Tuscan bean stew

- Chicken and baked potatoes with kale curry
- Kale and red onion with buckwheat

- Chinese-style pork with Pak Choi

- Salmon sirt super salad

- Smoked salmon pasta with chili and arugula

- Fragrant Asian hotpot

- Sesame chicken salad

- King prawns stir-fried with buckwheat noodles

- Mushroom soup

- Backed chicken breast with walnuts, pesto, and red onion salad

- Baked potatoes with spicy chickpea stew

- The green juice salad

Feel free to go online and find all sorts of Sirtfood recipes. Make your own choices, get original, and enjoy!

Snacks

Well, when it comes to snacks, we talk about rewards or a simple way to ensure our will to go along with a diet. The less we get the best it goes, but don't worry if you get two treats a day.

Sirtfood snacks will give your cells an extra help in the sirtuin activation process.

Let's see! We can indulge in fresh bites of fruits or vegetables we love, but we can indulge in desserts. Sirt ones, of course!

Here are some of my ideas, besides coffee and dark chocolate:

- Raspberry and blackcurrant jelly

- Chocolate cupcakes with matcha icing

- Matcha with vanilla

- Date and walnut cinnamon bites

- Fresh fruits(strawberries, apples, and oranges)

- Celery and hummus

Drinks

In these two weeks of the second phase, we can use other beverages too. Always for the variety!

Except for green juice, water, tea, coffee, cocoa, milk, and red wine, we can expand our choice to:

- Kale and blackcurrant smoothie

- Green tea smoothie

- Turmeric tea

- Grape and melon juice, and so on.

Please feel free to try any combination of your favorite fruits and vegetables!

You will get used to the spicy flavors of some ingredients, but you will most importantly benefit from the most nutrient properties of Sirtfoods.

Keep up the excellent work!

Sirtfood Diet recipes

I came up with a list of the most popular recipes of the Sirtfood Diet. These are the most used by celebrities and other people. They range from main courses to desserts and smoothies.

In the second phase of the diet, you can mix them the way you want, so you vary your meals and don't get bored with the same stuff every day.

Enjoy!

1. CHICKEN SALAD

The chicken salad is the coronation of the Sirtfood Diet. It is easy to make and healthy for lunch or dinner.

Ingredients:

- 75 g natural yogurt
- juice of 1/4 of a lemon
- 1 tsp. chopped coriander
- 1 tsp. of ground turmeric
- 1/2 tsp. of mild curry powder
- 100 g cooked chicken breast(bite-sized pieces cut)
- 6 chopped walnut halves
- 1 Medjool date, finely chopped
- 20 g diced red onion
- 1 Bird's eye chili
- 40 g arugula, to serve

Instructions:

Mix the yogurt, the lemon juice, coriander, and spices in a large bowl. Now add all the remaining ingredients and serve on a bed of rocket.

2. KING PRAWN STIR FRY WITH BUCKWHEAT NOODLES

Ingredients:

- 300 g buckwheat or soba noodles
- 2 tbsp. extra virgin olive oil
- 1 red onion thinly sliced
- 2 sliced sticks of celery
- 100 g kale roughly chopped
- 100 g green beans
- 3 cm of grated ginger
- 3 grated or chopped garlic cloves

- 1 Bird's eye chili seeds (the membranes removed and finely chopped)
- 600 g king prawns
- 2 tbsp. tamari/soy sauce plus extra for serving
- 2 tbsp. parsley, chopped

Instructions:

- Cook the noodles for 3-5 minutes. Drain and rinse in cold water. Drizzle over olive oil, mix and put aside.
- In the meantime, you can prepare the other ingredients.
- In a large frying pan or wok, fry the red onion and the celery in olive oil over low heat for 3 minutes until soft, then add the kale and green beans. Now cook over medium-high heat for 3 minutes.

- Turn the heat down again, add the ginger, garlic, chili, and prawns. Fry until the prawns are hot all the way through.

- Add the noodles, tamari, or soy sauce and cook for one minute until the noodles are warm again. Sprinkle with parsley and serve.

3. KALE AND RED ONION DHAL WITH BUCKWHEAT

Delicious and very nutritious, it is easy to make. It is also naturally gluten-free, dairy-free, and vegetarian.

Ingredients:

- 1 tbsp. olive oil
- 1 sliced small red onion
- 3 grated garlic cloves
- 2 cm of grated ginger

- 1 birds eye chili (deseeded and chopped)

- 2 tsp. turmeric

- 2 tsp. garam masala

- 160 g red lentils

- 400 ml coconut milk

- 200 ml water

- 100 g kale (spinach is also an option)

- 160 g buckwheat/brown rice

Instructions:

- Put the olive oil in a large saucepan and add the onion. Cook on a low heat for 5 minutes until softened.

- Add the garlic, ginger, and chili. Now cook for one more minute.

- Add the turmeric, the garam masala, and a splash of water. Now cook for 1 more minute.

- Add the red lentils, coconut milk, and 200ml water, merely filling the coconut milk can with water and then tipping it into the saucepan.

- Mix everything thoroughly and cook for 20 minutes over a gentle heat. Stir occasionally. Add a little more water only if the dhal starts to stick.

- After 20 minutes, add the kale, stir thoroughly, and cook for another 5 minutes.

- About 15 minutes before the curry is ready, place the buckwheat in a saucepan and add boiling water. Now cook for an extra 10 minutes. Drain the buckwheat and serve with the dhal.

4. CHICKEN, BROCCOLI AND BEETROOT SALAD WITH AVOCADO PESTO

This superfood is packed with ingredients to give your body a boost, such as red onion, nigella seeds, walnuts, and lemon.

Ingredients:

- 250g thin-stemmed broccoli
- 2 tsp of rapeseed oil
- 3 skinless chicken breasts
- 1 thinly sliced red onion
- 100g watercress
- 2 raw beetroots (peeled and julienned)
- 1 tsp nigella seeds
- For the avocado pesto:
- 1 small pack of basil
- 1 avocado
- 1/2 crushed garlic cloves

- 25g crumbled walnut halves

- 1 tbsp of rapeseed oil

- juice and zest from one lemon

Instructions:

- Bring a medium pan of water to the boil, add the broccoli and cook for 2 minutes. Drain and refresh under cold water.

- Now, heat a griddle pan, toss the broccoli in 1/2 tsp of the rapeseed oil, and cook for 2-3 mins, often turning until a little charred. Let it cool.

- Brush the chicken with the remaining oil and season as you like. Grill for 3-4 mins each side, until well cooked through.

- Let it cool, and slice or shred into chunky pieces.

- Next, make the pesto. Pick the leaves from the basil and put aside a handful for the salad. Put the rest in the small bowl of a food processor. Add the flesh from the avocado to the food processor with the garlic, walnuts, the oil, 1 tbsp lemon juice, 2-3 tbsp of cold water, and some seasoning. Mix until smooth, then transfer to a serving dish. Pour the remaining lemon juice over the onions and let it sit for a few minutes.

- Pile the watercress onto a large platter. Toss through the broccoli and onion, along with the lemon juice. Top with the beetroot, but don't mix it in, and the chicken. Scatter over the remaining basil leaves, the lemon zest, and nigella seeds. Now serve with the avocado pesto.

5. KALE WITH LEMON TAHINI DRESSING

A quick stir-fried side dish. The lemon tahini dressing is for a flavourful and fresh way to enjoy your greens.

Ingredients:

- juice of a lemon
- 1 crushed garlic clove
- 50g tahini
- 1 tbsp olive oil
- 200g kale

Instructions:

- Make the dressing. Put the lemon juice, the garlic, tahini, and 50ml of cold water in a bowl. Mix well to form a loose dressing, then season to taste.

- Heat the oil in a frying pan and stir-fry the kale for 3 mins. Now add half the dressing to the pan and cook for a further 30 secs. Transfer into a serving bowl and drizzle over the remaining dressing.

6. BUNLESS BEEF BURGERS WITH ALL THE TRIMMINGS

Who wouldn't enjoy an excellent burger with sweet potato fries?

Ingredients:

- 125 g lean minced beef (5% fat)
- 15 g finely chopped red onion
- 1 tsp. chopped parsley
- 1 tsp. extra virgin olive oil
- 150 g sweet potatoes
- 1 tsp. extra virgin olive oil

- 1 tsp. dried rosemary

- 1 unpeeled garlic clove

- 10 g Cheddar cheese (sliced or grated)

- 150 g red onion, sliced into rings

- 30 g of sliced tomato

- 10 g rocket

- 1 gherkin (optional)

Instructions:

- Heat the oven to 428°F.

- Start by making the fries. Peel then cut the sweet potatoes into chips. Toss them with olive oil, rosemary, and garlic. Place them on a baking sheet then roast for at least 30 minutes or until nice and crispy.

- For the burger, mix the onion and parsley with the minced beef. Use your hands.

- Heat a frying pan over medium heat, add the olive oil, and place the burger on one side of the pan. Add the onion rings on the other side. Now cook the burger for 6 minutes on each side. Now, fry the onion rings.
- When the burger is ready, top it with the cheese and red onion. Top with the tomato, rocket, and gherkin(if you wish). Serve with the fries.

7. CHICKEN SKEWERS WITH SATAY SAUCE

A minimal effort main course, full of flavor and spice.

Ingredients:
- 150 g chicken breast (cut into chunks)
- 1 tsp. ground turmeric

- 1/2 tsp. of extra virgin olive oil

- 50 g buckwheat

- 30 g Kale (stalks removed and sliced)

- 30 g sliced celery

- 4 chopped walnut halves

- 20 g diced red onion

- 1 chopped garlic clove

- 1 tsp. extra virgin olive oil

- 1 tsp. curry powder

- 1 tsp. Of ground turmeric

- 50 ml chicken stock

- 150 ml Coconut milk

- 1 tbsp. walnut or peanut butter

- 1 tbsp. chopped coriander

Instructions:

- Mix the chicken with turmeric and olive oil.

Now set aside to marinate (at least 30 minutes).

- Cook the buckwheat according to the instructions. Add the kale and celery for the last 5–7 minutes of the cooking time and drain it.

- Now set up the grill on high heat.

- For the sauce, gently fry the red onion and garlic in the olive oil for 2 or 3 minutes. Add the spices and keep cooking for a further minute. Add the stock and coconut milk, then bring to the boil. Now add the walnut butter and stir through. Reduce the heat and simmer the sauce until creamy and rich(8 or 10 minutes).

- In the meantime, thread the chicken onto the skewers, place them on the hot grill for 10 minutes, turning them after 5 minutes.

- To serve, stir the coriander through the sauce and pour it over the skewers. Now scatter over the chopped walnuts and serve.

8. SMOKED SALMON OMELETTE

A ⬚uick and easy Sirtfood dish packed with flavor.

Ingredients:

- 2 medium eggs
- 100 g sliced smoked salmon
- 1/2 tsp. Capers
- 10 g chopped arugula
- 1 tsp. chopped parsley
- 1 tsp. of extra virgin olive oil

Instructions:

- Crack the eggs into a bowl and whisk them well. Add the salmon, capers, arugula, and parsley.
- Heat the olive oil in a frying pan until hot but not smoking. Add the egg mixture and, with a

spatula, move the mixture around the pan until it is even. Reduce the heat and let it cook through. Slide the spatula around the edges and fold the omelet in half.

9. SHAKSHUKA

A healthy recipe of spicy baked eggs and kale!

Ingredients:

- 1 tsp. extra virgin olive oil
- 40 g finely chopped red onion
- 1 chopped garlic clove
- 30 g celery, finely chopped
- 1 Bird's eye chili, finely chopped
- 1 tsp. ground cumin
- 1 tsp. ground turmeric
- 1 tsp. of paprika
- 400 g chopped tomatoes

- 30 g Kale (stems removed and chopped)

- 1 tbsp. chopped parsley

- 2 medium eggs

Instructions:

- Heat a frying pan over medium-low heat. Add the oil and fry the onion, garlic, celery, chili, and spices for 1 or 2 minutes.

- Add the tomatoes, then leave the sauce to simmer for 20 minutes, stirring occasionally.

10. DATE AND WALNUT PORRIDGE

The ultimate Sirtfood breakfast !

Ingredients:

- 200 ml milk or soy milk

- 1 Medjool date, chopped

- 35 g buckwheat flakes

- 1 tsp. walnut butter or 4 chopped walnut halves

- 50 g hulled strawberries

Instructions:

- Place the milk and Medjool date in a pan and heat gently; then add the buckwheat flakes and cook until the porridge has the desired consistency.

- Stir in the walnut butter(walnuts), and top with the strawberries.

- Add the kale and cook for a further 5 minutes. If the sauce is getting too thick, add a little water. When your sauce has a creamy consistency, add in the parsley.

- Make two little wells in the sauce and crack the eggs into them. Reduce the heat and cover the pan with a lid. Let the eggs cook for 10–12 minutes. If you prefer the yolks to be firm, cook for extra 3 or 4 minutes. Serve immediately.

11. BRAISED PUY LENTILS

This roasted recipe is full of flavor.

Ingredients:

- 8 halved Cherry tomatoes

- 2 tsp. extra virgin olive oil

- 40 g thinly sliced red onion

- 1 chopped garlic clove

- 40 g celery, thinly sliced

- 40 g carrots (peeled and sliced)

- 1 tsp. paprika

- 1 tsp. thyme

- 75 g Puy lentils

- 220 ml vegetable stock

- 50 g chopped Kale

- 1 tbsp. chopped parsley

- 20 g arugula

Instructions:

- Heat your oven to 248°F.

- Put the tomatoes into a roasting tin in the oven for 35–45 minutes.

- Heat a saucepan over low–medium heat. Add one teaspoon of the olive oil with the red onion, garlic, celery, and carrot and fry for 1–2 minutes. Add in the paprika and thyme, then cook for a further minute.

- Rinse the lentils in a sieve, then add them to the pan along with the stock. Bring to the boil and reduce the heat. Now simmer gently for 20 minutes with a lid on it. Stir the pan every 7 minutes, adding a little water only if the level drops too much.

- Add the kale and keep cooking for a further 10 minutes. When the lentils are ready, stir in the parsley and the roasted tomatoes. Drizzle the rocket with the remaining teaspoon of olive oil and serve.

12. PRAWN ARRABBIATA

Ingredients:

- 125-150 g raw or cooked prawns (king prawns)
- 65 g buckwheat pasta
- 1tbsp extra virgin olive oil

- For arrabbiata sauce:
- 40 g finely chopped red onion
- 1 chopped garlic clove
- 30 g celery, finely chopped

- 1 Bird's eye chili, finely chopped

- 1 tsp dried mixed herbs

- 1 tsp extra virgin olive oil

- 2 tbsp white wine (if you wish)

- 400 g tinned chopped tomatoes

- 1 tbsp chopped parsley

Instructions:

- Fry the onion, garlic, celery, chili, and dried herbs in the oil over medium-low heat for 1–2 minutes. Turn the heat up to medium, then add the wine and cook for another minute. Now add the tomatoes and leave the sauce to simmer over medium-low heat for 20–30 minutes, until it has a creamy consistency.

- In the meantime, bring a pan of water to the boil, then cook the pasta according to instructions. When cooked, drain, toss with the olive oil and keep in the pan until needed.

- If you are using raw prawns, add them to the sauce and cook it all for a further 3–4 minutes until they have turned pink, then add the parsley and serve. When using cooked prawns, com them with the parsley, bring the sauce to the boil, and serve.

- Add the cooked pasta to the sauce, mix it all thoroughly and serve.

13. TURMERIC BAKED SALMON

An easy to do and healthy course that is full of Eastern spice!

Ingredients:

- 1 skinned salmon

- 1 tsp. extra virgin olive oil

- 1 tsp. ground turmeric

- 1/4 juice of a lemon

- 1 tsp. extra virgin olive oil

- 40 g finely chopped red onion

- 60 g tinned green lentils

- 1 chopped garlic clove

- 1 Bird's eye chili, finely chopped

- 150 g celery, cut into 2cm lengths

- 1 tsp. mild curry powder

- 130 g tomato, cut into 8 wedges

- 100 ml chicken or vegetable stock

- 1 tbsp. chopped parsley

Instructions:

- Heat the oven to 392°F.

- Start with the celery. Heat a frying pan over medium-low heat, add the olive oil, then the onion, garlic, the ginger, chili, and spicy celery.

Fry gently until softened but not colored, then add the curry powder and keep cooking for a further minute.

• Add the tomatoes, the stock, and lentils and simmer gently for 10 minutes. Feel free to increase or decrease the cooking time, depending on how crunchy you like your celery.

• In the meantime, mix the turmeric, the oil, and lemon juice and rub over the salmon. Place it on a baking tray and cook for further 8 or 10 minutes.

• Now, stir the parsley through the celery and serve with the salmon.

14. EASY PEASY CHICKEN CURRY

Ingredients

- 1 red onion roughly chopped

- 3 garlic cloves roughly chopped

- 2 cm fresh ginger(peeled and chopped)

- 2 teaspoons of garam masala

- 2 teaspoons ground cumin

- 2 teaspoons of ground turmeric

- 1 cinnamon stick optional

- 6 cardamom pods(if you wish)

- 1 tablespoon olive oil

- 8 boneless skinless chicken thighs (or 4 chicken breasts), cut into bite-sized chunks

- 1 x 400ml tin coconut milk

- 2 tablespoons of chopped fresh coriander chopped

- 200 g buckwheat brown rice/basmati rice (for the serving)

Instructions:

- Place the onion, garlic, and the ginger in a food processor and blitz until it is a paste. You can also use a hand blender, or just chop the ingredients very finely and continue as below.

- Add the garam masala, cumin, and turmeric to the paste and stir it all together. Put it all aside.

- Next, put 1 tablespoon of olive oil in a deep pan. Heat the pan on high heat for one minute, then add the chopped up chicken thighs. Stir-fry the chicken on high heat for 2 minutes, then turn the heat down and add the curry paste. Allow the chicken to cook in the paste for 3 minutes and then add half the coconut milk (200ml), the cinnamon, and cardamom (if using). Bring to the boil and turn down and allow to simmer for 30 minutes until the curry sauce is thick!

• If the curry starts to get dry, simply add a splash more coconut milk. You may not need it all, but if you like a slightly more saucy curry, just add more!

• In the meantime, make your accompaniment (buckwheat or rice) and any side dishes.

• When the curry is ready, you can add the chopped coriander and serve it immediately with buckwheat or rice, and a nice glass of red wine!

15. BAKED POTATOES WITH SPICY CHICKPEA STEW (VEGAN)

This spicy Chickpea stew is delicious and makes an excellent topping for baked potatoes. It is also vegetarian, vegan, gluten-free, and dairy-free. And it contains chocolate!

Ingredients:

- 4-6 baking potatoes pricked all over
- 2 tablespoons of olive oil
- 2 finely chopped red onions
- 4 crushed garlic cloves
- 2 cm ginger grated
- 1 -2 teaspoons chili flakes
- 2 tablespoons of cumin seeds
- 2 tablespoons turmeric
- a splash of water
- 2 x 400g tins chopped tomatoes

- 2 tablespoons unsweetened cocoa powder

- 2 x 400g tins chickpeas (kidney beans, if you prefer)

- 2 yellow peppers (or whatever color you wish), chopped into bite-sized pieces

- 2 tablespoons of parsley(plus extra for garnish)

- salt and pepper to taste

- side salad (optional)

Instructions:

- Preheat the oven to 392°F. Meanwhile, prepare your ingredients.

- When the oven is hot enough, put your potatoes in the oven, and cook for 1 hour.

- Once the potatoes are in the oven, put the olive oil and chopped red onion in a wide saucepan, then cook gently, with the lid on for 5 minutes, until the onions are soft.

• Remove the lid; add the garlic, ginger, cumin, and chili. Now, cook for a further minute on low heat, then add the turmeric and a tiny splash of water. Now cook for another minute, making sure not to let the pan get too dry.

• Next, add in the tomatoes, cocoa powder, chickpeas (including the chickpea water), and yellow pepper. Bring to a boil, then simmer on a low heat for 45 minutes or until the sauce is thick. The stew should be done at the same time as the potatoes.

• Finally, stir in the 2 tablespoons of parsley, a bit of salt and pepper (if you wish), and serve the stew on top of the baked potatoes with a simple side salad if you want to.

16. KALE AND BLACKCURRANT SMOOTHIE

Ingredients:

- 2 tsp honey

- 1 cup freshly made green tea

- 10 baby kale leaves with stalks removed

- 1 ripe banana

- 40 g blackcurrants- washed and stalks removed

- 6 ice cubes

Instructions:

- Stir the honey into the warm tea until dissolved. Mix all the ingredients in a blender until smooth. Serve immediately.

17. BUCKWHEAT PASTA SALAD

Ingredients:

- 50g buckwheat pasta(cooked according to directions)
- a large handful of rocket
- a small handful of basil leaves
- 8 halved cherry tomatoes
- 1/2 avocado, diced
- 10 olives
- 1 tbsp extra virgin olive oil
- 20g pine nuts

Intructions:

- Gently combine all the ingredients, except for the pine nuts and arrange on a plate, then scatter the pine nuts over the top.

18. GREEK SALAD SKEWERS

Ingredients:

- 2 wooden skewers(best if pre-soaked in water for 30 minutes)
- 8 large black olives
- 8 cherry tomatoes
- 1 yellow pepper, cut into 8 squares
- 1/2 red onion (halved and separated into 8 piece
- 100g (about 10cm) cucumber, cut into 4 slices and halved
- 100g feta, cut into 8 cubes

For the dressing:

- 1 tbsp extra virgin olive oil
- the juice of ½ lemon
- 1 tsp balsamic vinegar

- 1/2 clove garlic, peeled and crushed
- a few leaves basil, finely chopped (or ½ tsp dried mixed herbs to replace basil and oregano)
- a few leaves oregano, finely chopped
- salt and freshly ground black pepper

Instructions:

- Thread each skewer with the salad ingredients: olive, tomato, yellow pepper, red onion, cucumber, feta, tomato, olive, yellow pepper, red onion, cucumber, and feta.
- Put all the dressing ingredients in a bowl and mix thoroughly. Pour over the skewers.

19. KALE, EDAMAME AND TOFU CURRY

Easy to keep either refrigerated or frozen for another day.

Serves: 4, Ready in 45 minutes

Ingredients:

- 1 tbsp of rapeseed oil
- 1 chopped large onion
- 4 grated cloves garlic
- 1 large thumb (7cm) ginger (peeled and grated)
- 1 red chili (deseeded and thinly sliced)
- 1/2 tsp of ground turmeric
- 1/4 tsp of cayenne pepper
- 1 tsp paprika
- 1/2 tsp ground cumin
- 1 tsp salt
- 250g dried red lentils

- 1 liter boiling water

- 50g frozen soy edamame beans

- 200g firm tofu, chopped into cubes

- 2 tomatoes, roughly chopped

- the juice of 1 lime

- 200g kale leaves (stalks removed and torn)

Instructions:

- Put the oil in a heavy-bottomed pan on low-medium heat. Then add the onion and cook for 5 minutes before adding the garlic, ginger, and chili and keep cooking for a further two minutes. Add the turmeric, cayenne, paprika, cumin, and salt. Stir through before adding the red lentils and stirring again.

- Pour in the boiling water, then bring to a hearty simmer for 10 minutes. Now reduce the heat and cook for a further 20-30 minutes until it has a thick consistency.

• Add the soya beans, tofu, and tomatoes and cook for a further 5 minutes. Add the lime juice and kale leaves and cook until the kale is just tender.

20. CHOCOLATE CUPCAKES WITH MATCHA ICING

Ingredients:

• 150g self-raising flour

• 200g caster sugar

• 60g cocoa

• ½ tsp salt

• ½ tsp fine espresso coffee

• 120ml milk

• ½ tsp vanilla extract

- 50ml vegetable oil

- 1 egg

- 120ml boiling water

For the icing:

- 50g butter, at room temperature

- 50g icing sugar

- 1 tbsp matcha green tea powder

- ½ tsp vanilla bean paste

- 50g soft cream cheese

Instructions:

- Preheat the oven to 356ºF. Line a cupcake tin with paper or use silicone cake cases.

- Place the flour, sugar, cocoa, salt, and espresso powder in a bowl and mix thoroughly.

- Now add the milk, vanilla extract, vegetable oil, and egg to the other ingredients, then use an electric mixer to beat until well combined. Carefully pour in the boiling water and beat on low speed until well combined. Next, use a high speed to beat for another minute so you add air to the batter.

• Spread the batter evenly in the cake cases. Each cake case should be ¾ full. Now, bake in the oven for 15-18 minutes, until the mixture bounces back when tapped. When is ready, remove from the oven and let it cool completely before icing.

• For the icing, cream the butter and icing sugar until it's pale and smooth, then add the matcha powder and vanilla and stir again. At the end, add the cream cheese and beat until smooth. Spread over the cakes and serve.

21. SESAME CHICKEN SALAD

Ingredients:

- 1 tbsp sesame seeds

- 1 cucumber (peeled, deseeded, and sliced)

- 100g baby kale, roughly chopped

- 60g Pak Choi, shredded

- ½ sliced red onion

- a large handful of chopped parsley

- 150g cooked chicken, shredded

For the dressing:

- 1 tbsp extra virgin olive oil

- 1 tsp sesame oil

- the juice of 1 lime

- 1 tsp clear honey

- 2 tsp of soy sauce

Instructions:

- First, toast the sesame seeds in a frying pan for at least 2 minutes or until lightly browned. Next, transfer to a plate and let it cool.

- In a bowl, mix the olive oil, sesame oil, lime juice, honey, and soy sauce for the dressing.

- Now, place the cucumber, kale, Pak Choi, red onion, and parsley in bowl and gently mix. Pour over the dressing and mix again.

- Arrange the salad on two plates and top with the shredded chicken, then sprinkle over the sesame seeds, and serve.

22. MUSHROOM SCRAMBLE EGGS

Ingredients:

* 2 eggs

* 1 tsp of ground turmeric

* 1 tsp mild curry powder

* 20g chopped kale

* 1 tsp of extra virgin olive oil

* ½ Bird's eye chilli, sliced

* a handful of sliced mushrooms

* 5g parsley, finely chopped

* seed mixture as a topper and Rooster Sauce
for flavor

Instructions:

* First, mix the turmeric and curry powder,
then add a little water until you have obtained a
light paste.

- Next, steam the kale for about 2– 3 minutes.

- Heat the oil in a frying pan over medium heat and fry the chilli with the mushrooms for 2– 3 minutes or until they are brown and soften.

23. AROMATIC CHICKEN BREAST WITH KALE, RED ONION, AND SALSA

Ingredients:

- 120g skinless and boneless chicken breast
- 2 tsp of ground turmeric
- the juice of ¼ lemon
- 1 tbsp of extra virgin olive oil
- 50g chopped kale
- 20g sliced red onion
- 1 tsp chopped fresh ginger
- 50g buckwheat

Instructions:

- For the salsa, remove the eye from the tomato, then chop it very finely, keeping as much of the li☐uid as possible. Now, mix with the chilli, capers, parsley, and the lemon juice.

- Heat the oven to 428°F. Now, marinate the chicken breast in 1 teaspoon of the turmeric, the lemon juice, and a lbit of oil. Let ir rest for 5 to 10 minutes.

- Next, heat an ovenproof frying pan until hot, then add the marinated chicken and cook for a minute on each side, until pale golden. Now, transfer to the oven for about 8–10 minutes or until well cooked. Remove from the oven, cover with foil, and let it rest for 5 minutes before serving.

- In the meantime, cook the kale in a steamer for 5 minutes, then fry the red onions and ginger in a little oil, just until soft but not coloured. Now, add the kale and fry for another minute.

• Cook the buckwheat according to instructions with the remaining teaspoon of turmeric. To be served with the chicken, vegetables, and salsa.

24. GREEN TEA SMOOTHIE

Matcha powder- a highly concentrated Japanese green tea, that we can find in specialist tea shops.

Ingredients:
• 2 ripe bananas
• 250 ml of milk
• 2 tsp Matcha green tea powder
• 1/2 tsp vanilla bean paste or seeds from a vanilla pod

- 6 ice cubes

- 2 tsp honey

Instructions:

- Blend all the ingredients in a blender and serve in two glasses.

25. SIRT FOOD MISO-MARINATED COD WITH STIR-FRIED GREENS AND SESAME

Ingredients:

- 20g miso

- 1 tbsp mirin

- 1 tbsp of extra virgin olive oil

- 200g skinless cod fillet

- 20g sliced red onion

- 40g sliced celery

- 1 chopped garlic clove

- 1 Bird's eye chili, chopped

- 1 tsp finely chopped fresh ginger

- 60g green beans

- 50g kale, roughly chopped

- 1 tsp of sesame seeds

- 5g chopped parsley

- 1 tbsp tamari

- 30g buckwheat

- 1 tsp ground turmeric

Instructions:

- First, mix the miso, mirin, and 1 teaspoon of oil. Rub it all over the cod and let it marinate for at least 30 minutes. Heat the oven to 428°F.

- Bake the cod for at least 10 minutes.

- In the meantime, heat a wok or frying pan with the remaining oil, then add in the onion and stir-fry for a few minutes. Now add the celery, garlic, chilli, ginger, green beans, and kale, then toss and fry until the kale is tender and well cooked. You may add a little water to the pan occasionally.

• Next, cook the buckwheat according to instructions with the turmeric for at least 3 minutes.

• Finally, add the sesame seeds, parsley, and tamari to the stir-fry. Serve with the greens and fish.

26.RASPBERRY AND BLACKCURRANT JELLY

It's best to make the jelly in advance so that it is ready to eat first thing in the morning.

Ingredients:
• 100g washed raspberries

- 2 leaves gelatine

- 100g blackcurrants (washed and stalks removed)

- 2 tbsp granulated sugar

- 300ml water

Instructions:

Arrange the raspberries in serving dishes or molds. Put the gelatine leaves into a bowl of water.

Put the blackcurrants in a pan with the sugar and 100ml water, then bring to the boil. Simmer vigorously for 5 minutes, then remove from the heat. Leave to stand for 2 minutes.

Squeeze out the excess water from the gelatine leaves, then add them to the saucepan. Stir until fully dissolved and the rest of the water. Pour the liquid into the prepared dishes and refrigerate. The jellies should be ready in about 3-4 hours.

27.APPLE PANCAKES WITH BLACKCURRANT COMPOTE

These pancakes are decadent but healthy!

Ingredients:

- 75g porridge oats

- 125g plain flour

- 1 tsp of baking powder

- 2 tbsp caster sugar

- a pinch of salt

- 2 apples (peeled, cored, and cut into tiny pieces)

- 300ml of semi-skimmed milk

- 2 egg whites

- 2 tsp light olive oil

For the compote:

- 120g blackcurrants (washed and stalks removed)
- 2 tbsp sugar
- 3 tbsp water

Instructions:

- First, make the compote. Now place the blackcurrants, sugar, and water in a small pan. Bring to a simmer, then cook for at least 10 minutes.
- Place the oats, flour, baking powder, sugar, and a pinch of salt in a large bowl and mix well. Now, stir in the apple, then whisk in the milk a little at a time until you have a smooth mixture. Whisk the egg whites to stiff peaks and then fold into the pancake batter. Transfer the batter to a jug.

- Heat 1/2 tsp oil in a frying pan on medium-high heat and pour in approximately a quarter of the batter. Cook on both sides until golden brown. Remove and repeat to make four pancakes.
- Serve the pancakes with blackcurrant compote drizzled on top.

28. FRUIT SALAD

Ingredients:
- ½ cup freshly made green tea
- 1 tsp honey
- 1 halved orange
- 1 apple, cored and roughly chopped
- 10 red seedless grapes
- 10 blueberries

Instructions:

- Stir the honey into half a cup of green tea, then add the juice of half the orange. Let it cool.
- Chop the other half of the orange and place it in a bowl with the chopped apple, grapes, and blueberries. Pour over the tea, then leave to steep for a few minutes before serving.

29. SIRTFOOD BITES

Ingredients:

- 120g walnuts
- 30g dark chocolate (broken into pieces), or cocoa nibs
- 250g pitted Medjool dates
- 1 tbsp cocoa powder
- 1 tbsp of ground turmeric
- 1 tbsp of extra virgin olive oil

- 1 tsp vanilla extract

- 1–2 tbsp of water

Instructions:

- Place the walnuts and chocolate in a food processor and blend until you obtain a fine powder.

- Add all the other ingredients except the water, then blend until the mixture forms a ball. Feel free to add some water depending on the consistency of the mixture -too sticky is not good!

- With your hands, form the mixture into bite-sized balls, refrigerate in an airtight container for at least one hour before serving.

- You could roll some of the balls in some more cocoa or coconut flakes to obtain a different finish if you like.

- You can keep them for up to one week in your fridge.

30. SIRT MUESLI

Ingredients:
- 20g buckwheat flakes
- 10g buckwheat puffs
- 15g coconut flakes or desiccated coconut
- 40g pitted and chopped Medjool dates
- 15g chopped walnuts
- 10g cocoa nibs
- 100g strawberries (hulled and chopped)
- 100g plain Greek yogurt (soy or coconut yogurt for vegans)

Instructions:

- Mix all of the ingredients, adding the yogurt and strawberries before serving if you are making it in bulk.

31. CHINESE-STYLE PORK WITH PAK CHOI

Ingredients:

- 400g firm tofu, cut into cubes
- 1 tbsp of cornflour
- 1 tbsp of water
- 125ml chicken stock
- 1 tbsp of rice wine
- 1 tbsp tomato purée
- 1 tsp of brown sugar
- 1 tbsp of soy sauce
- 1 crushed clove garlic

- 1 thumb (5cm) grated ginger

- 1 tbsp of rapeseed oil

- 100g sliced shiitake mushrooms

- 1 shallot, peeled and sliced

- 200g sliced Pak Choi or Choi sum, and 400g pork mince

- 100g beansprouts

- a large handful of chopped parsley

Instructions:

- Arrange the tofu on kitchen paper, cover with more kitchen paper and put aside.

- In a bowl, mix the cornflour and water, making sure to remove all lumps. Now, add the chicken stock, rice wine, tomato purée, sugar, and soy sauce, then add the crushed garlic and ginger and stir together.

• In a wok or large frying pan, heat the oil to a high temperature, then add the shiitake mushrooms and stir-fry for at least 3 minutes or until cooked and glossy. Now, remove the mushrooms from the pan and set aside. Next, add the tofu to the pan and stir-fry until golden on all sides, then remove with a slotted spoon and put aside.

• Next, add the shallot and Pak Choi to the wok, stir-fry for 2 minutes, then add the mince. Keep cooking until the mince is well cooked, then add the sauce, reduce the heat a notch and allow the sauce to bubble round the meat for two minutes. Finally, add the beansprouts, shiitake mushrooms, and tofu to the pan and warm through. Remove from the heat, spread the parsley on top and serve immediately.

32. TUSCAN BEAN STEW

Ingredients:

- 1 tbsp extra virgin olive oil
- 50g red onion, finely chopped
- 30g carrot, peeled and finely chopped
- 30g celery, trimmed and finely chopped
- 1 garlic clove, finely chopped
- 1/2 Bird's eye chili, finely chopped (optional)
- 1 tsp herbes de Provence
- 200ml vegetable stock
- 1 x 400g tin chopped Italian tomatoes
- 1 tsp tomato purée
- 200g tinned mixed beans
- 50g kale, roughly chopped
- 1 tbsp roughly chopped parsley
- 40g buckwheat

Instructions:

- Place the oil in a saucepan over low–medium heat and fry the onion, carrot, celery, garlic, chili, and herbs, until the onion is soft but not brown colored.
- Add the stock, the tomato purée, and tomatoes and bring all to the boil. Now add the beans and let it simmer for 30 minutes.
- Add the kale and keep cooking for another 5–10 minutes, then add the parsley.
- Meanwhile, cook the buckwheat according to instructions, drain, and then serve with the stew.

33. SALMON SIRT SUPER SALAD

Ingredients:

- 50g of rocket

- 50g chicory leaves

- 100g smoked salmon slices (lentils, cooked chicken breast or tinned tuna)

- 80g avocado, peeled, stoned and sliced

- 40g celery, sliced

- 20g of sliced red onion

- 15g chopped walnuts

- 1 tbs capers

- 1 large Medjool date (pitted and chopped)

- 1 tbs extra-virgin olive oil

- the juice of ¼ lemon

- 10g parsley, chopped

- 10g lovage or celery leaves, chopped

Instructions:

- Place the salad leaves on a plate. Mix the remaining ingredients and serve on top of the leaves.

34.ASIAN SHRIMP STIR-FRY WITH BUCKWHEAT NOODLES

Ingredients:

- 1⁄3 pound (150g) shelled raw jumbo shrimp, deveined
- 2 teaspoons tamari (soy sauce-if you are not avoiding gluten)
- 2 teaspoons of extra virgin olive oil
- 3 ounces (75g) soba (buckwheat noodles)
- 2 chopped garlic cloves
- 1 Thai chili, finely chopped
- 1 teaspoon finely chopped ginger

- 1/8 cup (20g) slices of red onions

- 1/2 cup (45g) celery (trimmed and sliced, with leaves set aside)

- 1/2 cup (75g) green beans, chopped

- 3/4 cup (50g) chopped kale

- 1/2 cup (100ml) chicken stock

Instructions:

- Heat a frying pan and cook the shrimp in 1 teaspoon of the tamari and 1 teaspoon of the oil for at least 2 minutes.

- Next put the shrimp onto a plate. Wipe the pan out with a paper towel, since you're going to use it again.

- Now cook the noodles in boiling water for 5 -8 minutes or as directed on the package. Drain and put aside.

- Meanwhile, fry the garlic, chili, ginger, red onion, celery, green beans, and kale in the remaining tamari and oil over medium-high heat for at least 2 minutes. Next, add the stock and bring to a boil, then simmer for a minute or two, until the vegetables are cooked.

- Next, add the shrimp, noodles, and celery leaves to the pan, bring back to a boil, and remove from the heat and serve.

35.STRAWBERRY BUCKWHEAT TABBOULEH

Ingredients:

- 1/3 cup (50g) buckwheat
- 1 tablespoon ground turmeric
- 1/2 cup (80g) avocado
- 3/8 cup (65g) tomato

- 1/8 cup (20g) red onion

- 1/8 cup (25g) Medjool dates, pitted

- 1 tablespoon capers

- 3/4 cup (30g) parsley

- 2/3 cup (100g) strawberries, hulled

- 1 tablespoon extra virgin olive oil

- the juice of 1/2 lemon

- 1 ounce (30g) arugula

Instructions:

- Cook the buckwheat with the turmeric according to instructions.

- Drain and put aside to cool.

- Finely chop the avocado, tomato, red onion, dates, capers, and parsley and mix with the cooled buckwheat.

- Slice the strawberries and gently mix into the salad with the lemon juice and oil. Serve on a bed of arugula.

36. MATCHA WITH VANILLA

It's easy to make, and it only takes five minutes!

Ingredients:

- ½ tsp Matcha powder
- seeds from half a vanilla pod

Instructions:

- Boil the kettle, pour 100ml of the water into a measuring jug. Pour half the hot water into a bowl, to warm it, and add the Matcha powder and vanilla seeds.
- Whisk the mixture with a bamboo match until it's smooth, lump-free, and slightly bubbly.

Discard the water in the warmed tea bowl, and pour in the prepared Matcha tea.

37. TURMERIC TEA

This bright orange spice is popping up on menus in every corner of the world!

Ingredients:

- 3 heaped tsp of ground turmeric
- 1 tbsp grated ginger
- 1 small orange
- honey or agave and lemon slices (to serve)

Instructions:

- Boil 500ml water in the kettle. Place the turmeric, ginger, and orange zest into a teapot. Pour over the boiling water and let it infuse for around 5 mins.

- Drain through a sieve or tea strainer into two cups, add a slice of lemon and sweeten with honey or agave if you want.

38. DATE AND WALNUT CINNAMON BITES

Ingredients:

- 3 walnut halves
- 3 pitted Medjool dates
- a sprinkle of ground cinnamon, to taste

Instructions:

- Carefully cut each walnut half into three slices and do the same with the dates. Carefully place a slice of walnut on top of each Medjool date, then dust with cinnamon and serve.

39. RED CHICORY, PEAR, AND HAZELNUT SALAD

Ingredients:

- 2 heads of red or white chicory
- 2 ripe red Williams pears a good handful of rocket leaves
- 25g hazelnuts, toasted and chopped

For the dressing:

- 1 tsp green peppercorns in brine, optional
- 2 tbsp hazelnut or olive oil
- 2 tbsp mild salad oil
- 1 tsp sherry or cider vinegar

Instructions:

- Make the dressing. If using green peppercorns, lightly crush them in a bowl. Mix in the oils and vinegar, then add salt to taste.

- Trim away the chicory stalk ends and discard any limp or tired outer leaves. Carefully separate the leaves and arrange 5-6 on four plates.

- Remove the stalks from the pears and quarter the pears lengthways. Cut out the cores, then thinly slice the fruit. Place the pear slices on top of the chicory leaves, then spoon over half the dressing. Pour the remaining dressing over the rocket, then season with salt and pepper. Give the leaves a quick toss and pile on top of each salad. Next, sprinkle with the nuts and serve.

40. ITALIAN KALE

Ingredients:

- 3 tbsp olive oil

- 3 garlic cloves, finely sliced

- 3 tbsp red wine vinegar

- 300g cavolo nero or kale, roughly shredded

Instructions:

- Heat the oil in a large pan and sizzle the garlic, then add the vinegar and a splash of water.

- Tip the kale into the pan, cover, and wilt in the steam for 4-5 minutes. When the kale is wilted, season with a little sea salt.

41. BROCCOLI AND KALE GREEN SOUP

Ingredients:

- 500ml stock, made by mixing 1 tbsp of bouillon powder and boiling water in a jug
- 1 tbsp of sunflower oil
- 2 sliced garlic cloves
- 1 sliced thumb-sized piece ginger
- ½ tsp ground coriander
- 3cm/1in piece of grated fresh turmeric root
- ½ tsp of pink Himalayan salt
- 200g courgettes, roughly sliced
- 85g broccoli
- 100g chopped kale
- 1 lime, zested and juiced
- 1 small pack parsley, roughly chopped, reserving a few whole leaves to serve

Instructions:

- Put the oil in a pan, add the garlic, ginger, coriander, turmeric, and salt, then fry on medium heat for 2 mins. Now add 3 tbsp water to give a bit more moisture to the spices.

- Add the courgettes and continue cooking for 3 mins. Add 400ml stock and let it simmer for 3 mins.

- Now add the broccoli, kale, and lime juice. Keep cooking for another 3-4 minutes.

- Take off the heat, then add the chopped parsley. Pour everything into a blender and blend until smooth. Now garnish with lime zest and parsley.

42. STRAWBERRY, TOMATO AND WATERCRESS SALAD WITH HONEY & PINK PEPPER DRESSING

Ingredients:

- 300g strawberries
- 250g mixed tomatoes
- 100g watercress, woody stalks discarded

For the dressing:

- 1 tbsp pink peppercorns
- 2 strawberries (about 40g), chopped
- 1/2 tbsp honey
- 1/2 lemon, juiced
- 3 tbsp extra virgin olive oil

Instructions:

- Start with the dressing- toast the peppercorns in a dry frying pan for 1-2 minutes, then bash briefly with a pinch of salt. Add the strawberries and mash them to a paste.

- Next stir in the honey and lemon juice. Place the dressing into a bowl, and whisk in the olive oil. Now check for seasoning, then add a little more salt or lemon juice if you want. For the salad, cut the strawberries into quarters or slim wedges, and roughly chop the tomatoes, slicing or halving some. Mix with the watercress in the bowl.

- Finally arrange the salad onto four plates or pile onto a platter. Now spoon over any dressing left.

43. ORIENTAL SALMON AND BROCCOLI TRAYBAKE

Ingredients:

- 4 skin-on salmon fillets

- 1 head broccoli, broken into florets

- the juice ½ lemon and ½ lemon quartered

- a small bunch spring onions, sliced

- 2 tbsp of soy sauce

Instructions:

- First heat the oven to 356ºF. Put the salmon in a large roasting tin, leaving a bit of space between each fillet.

- Wash and drain the broccoli and arrange it in the tray around the fillets. Pour the lemon juice over and add the lemon quarters.

- Top with half the onions, then drizzle with a little olive oil and put in the oven for a least 14 minutes. Remove from the oven, sprinkle with the soy, then return to the oven for 4 minutes more, until the salmon is cooked through. Sprinkle with the remaining onions and serve.

44. SUPERHEALTHY SALMON SALAD

Ingredients:

- 100g couscous
- 1 tbsp olive oil
- 2 salmon fillets
- 200g sprouting broccoli (roughly shredded and larger stalks removed)
- the juice of 1 lemon
- seeds from half a pomegranate
- a small handful of pumpkin seeds

- 2 handfuls watercress

- olive oil and extra lemon wedges

Instructions:

- Bring water to a boil in a steamer. Now season the couscous and toss with 1 tsp oil. Pour the boiling water over the couscous, so it covers it by 1cm, then put aside. When the water comes to the boil, just tip the broccoli in, then lay the salmon in the tier above. Now cook for 3 minutes or until the salmon is well cooked through and the broccoli still tender. Next, drain the broccoli and run it under cold water.

- Now mix the remaining lemon juice and oil; toss the broccoli, pomegranate seeds, and pumpkin seeds in the couscous along with the lemon dressing. Finally, roughly chop the watercress and toss it through the couscous.

Serve with the salmon, and lemon wedges for squeezing over and extra olive oil for drizzling, if you want.

45. MALABAR PRAWNS

Malabar prawns- a specialty of the South Indian coast. Quick and very easy to prepare and full of exotic flavors!

Ingredients:

- 400g raw king prawns
- 2 tsp turmeric
- 3-4 tsp Kashmiri chili powder
- 4 tsp lemon juice (plus a squeeze)
- 40g ginger (half peeled and grated, the other half finely sliced into matchsticks)
- 1 tbsp vegetable oil
- 4 curry leaves

- 2-4 green chilies (halved and deseeded)

- 1 finely sliced onion

- 1 tsp cracked black pepper

- 40g fresh coconut, grated

- 1/2 small bunch of coriander leaves

Instructions:

- Rinse the prawns and pat dry. Toss them with the turmeric, chili powder, lemon juice, and grated ginger, then put aside.

- Heat the oil in a pan and add the curry leaves, chili, sliced ginger, and onion. Now cook for about 10 mins and add the black pepper.

- Thos the prawns in with any marinade, then stir-fry until cooked, for at least 2 minutes. If required, season and add a squeeze of lemon juice. Serve with the coconut and coriander leaves sprinkled on top.

46. CHICKEN, KALE AND SPROUT STIR-FRY

Brussels sprouts are not just for Christmas- add them to a fresh noodle pot for extra nutrition!

Ingredients:

- 100g soba noodle
- 100g shredded curly kale
- 2 tsp of sesame oil
- 2 lean chicken breasts (skin removed, sliced into thin strips)
- 25g piece fresh ginger, sliced into matchsticks
- 1 red pepper, thinly sliced
- a handful Brussels sprout, cut into quarters
- 1 tbsp soy sauce
- 2 tbsp white wine vinegar or rice wine
- the zest and juice of 1 lime

Instructions:

• Cook the noodles following the pack instructions, drain, and put aside. In the meantime, heat a frying pan or wok, add the kale along with a good splash of water, and cook for 1-2 minutes, until wilted, then cool under running water to keep the color.

• Add half the oil, then cook the chicken strips until browned. Now remove and put aside. Heat the remaining oil, fry the ginger, pepper, and sprouts until softened a little. Next, add the chicken, kale, and the noodles.

• Finally tip in the soy, rice wine, the lime zest, juice, and enough water to create a sauce, and serve immediately.

47. THE GREEN JUICE SALAD

An alternative to the Sirtfood green juice, this salad includes all the same ingredients as the green juice plus 2 additional Sirtfoods: walnuts and olive oil. Delicious and very easy to make!

Ingredients:

- juice of ½ lemon
- 1 cm ginger grated
- salt and pepper to taste
- 1 tablespoon olive oil
- 2 handfuls of sliced kale
- 1 handful rocket
- 1 tablespoon parsley
- 2 celery sticks sliced
- 1/2 green apple sliced
- 6 walnut halves

Instructions:

- Put the lemon juice, ginger, salt, pepper, and olive oil in a jam jar and shake to combine.

- Place the kale in a bowl and pour over the dressing. Stir the dressing into the kale for 1 minute.

- Add the other ingredients and mix them all.

48. TURMERIC CHICKEN AND KALE SALAD WITH HONEY LIME DRESSING

Notes: Chicken can be replaced with beef mince, fish, or chopped prawns. Vegetarians could use quinoa or chopped mushrooms.

Ingredients:

- For the chicken:
- 1 tsp. ghee or 1 tbsp coconut oil
- 1/2 medium brown onion

- 250-300 g / 9 oz. chicken mince or diced chicken thighs
- 1 large garlic clove
- 1 teaspoon turmeric powder
- 1 teaspoon of lime zest
- the juice of ½ lime
- 1/2 teaspoon salt and pepper

For the salad:
- 6 broccolini stalks /2 cups of broccoli florets
- 2 tablespoons of pumpkin seeds
- 3 large kale leaves, chopped and stems removed
- 1/2 sliced avocado
- a handful of chopped fresh coriander leaves
- a handful of chopped fresh parsley leaves

For the dressing:

- 3 tablespoons of lime juice

- 1 small, grated garlic clove

- 3 tablespoons extra-virgin olive oil

- 1 teaspoon raw honey

- 1/2 teaspoon Dijon mustard

- 1/2 teaspoon of sea salt and pepper

Instructions:

- Heat the ghee or coconut oil in a frying pan over medium-high heat. Now add the onion and sauté on medium heat for about 4-5 minutes or until golden. Now add the chicken mince and garlic and stir for another 2-3 minutes over medium-high heat.

- Next, add the turmeric, lime zest, lime juice, salt, and pepper and cook for a further 3-4 minutes. Set the mince aside.

- While the chicken is cooking, bring a saucepan of water to boil, then add the broccolini and cook for 2 minutes. Rinse under cold water, then cut into 3-4 pieces each.

- Add the pumpkin seeds to the pan and toast over medium heat for 2 minutes. Now, season with salt and put aside. You may also use raw pumpkin seeds.

- Place the chopped kale in a large bowl and pour over the dressing. Now toss the kale with the dressing, to soften the kale, kind of like what citrus juice does to fish or beef carpaccio.

- Finally, add the cooked chicken, broccolini, fresh herbs, pumpkin seeds, and avocado slices.

49.BUCKWHEAT NOODLES WITH CHICKEN, KALE, AND MISO DRESSING

Ingredients:

For the noodles:

- 2-3 handfuls of kale leaves (roughly cut)
- 150 g / 5 oz buckwheat noodles
- 3-4 sliced shiitake mushrooms
- 1 teaspoon coconut oil or ghee
- 1 brown onion, finely diced
- 1 medium free-range chicken breast, sliced
- 1 long red chili, thinly sliced
- 2 large garlic cloves, finely diced
- 2-3 tablespoons Tamari sauce

For the miso dressing:

- 1½ tablespoon of fresh organic miso
- 1 tablespoon of Tamari sauce

- 1 tablespoon of extra-virgin olive oil

- 1 tablespoon lemon or lime juice

- 1 teaspoon sesame oil

Instructions:

- Bring a saucepan of water to boil, then add the kale and cook for 1 minute. Now remove and put aside but reserve the water and bring it back to the boil. Add the soba noodles and cook according to instructions (about 5 minutes). Now rinse under cold water and put aside.

- In the meantime, fry the shiitake mushrooms in a pan with little ghee or coconut oil for about 2 minutes, just until lightly browned on each side. Sprinkle with sea salt and put aside.

- In the same pan, heat more coconut oil or ghee over medium-high heat. Sauté the onion and chili for 2-3 minutes, then add the chicken pieces. Cook for 5 minutes over medium heat, stirring occasionally, then add the garlic, tamari sauce, and a splash of water. Cook for a further 2 minutes until the chicken is well cooked through.

• Finally, add the kale and soba noodles and toss with the chicken.

• Mix the miso dressing, then drizzle over the noodles right at the end of cooking. In this way, you will keep all those beneficial probiotics in the miso alive and active.

50. CHOC CHIP GRANOLA

Chocolate at breakfast! Make sure to serve with a cup of green tea to give you plenty of sirtuins.

Ingredients:

• 200g jumbo oats

- 50g pecans, roughly chopped

- 3 tbsp light olive oil

- 20g butter

- 1 tbsp dark brown sugar

- 2 tbsp rice malt syrup

- 60g good-quality (70%) dark chocolate chips

Instructions:

- Preheat the oven to 320°F. Line a baking tray with a silicone sheet or baking parchment.

- Mix the oats and pecans in a bowl. In a small pan, gently heat the olive oil, butter, brown sugar, and rice malt syrup until the sugar and syrup have dissolved. Do not let it boil. Next, pour the syrup over the oats and stir thoroughly until the oats are fully covered.

- Spread the granola over the tray, spreading right into the corners. Leave clumps of the mixture with spacing. Now, bake in the oven for 20 minutes or until tinged golden brown at the edges. Next, remove from the oven and leave to cool completely.

• When cool, mix in the chocolate chips, then pour the granola into a jar. The granola will keep for at least 2 weeks.

51.BAKED SALMON SALAD WITH CREAMY MINT DRESSING

Ingredients:

• 1 salmon fillet (130g)

• 40g mixed salad leaves

• 40g young spinach leaves

• 2 radishes, trimmed and thinly sliced

• 5cm piece (50g) cucumber, cut into chunks

• 2 spring onions, trimmed and sliced

- 1 small handful (10g) parsley, roughly chopped

For the dressing:

- 1 tsp low-fat mayonnaise
- 1 tbsp natural yogurt
- 1 tbsp rice vinegar
- 2 leaves mint, finely chopped
- salt and ground black pepper

Instructions:

- Preheat the oven to 392°F.
- Place the salmon fillet on a baking tray, then bake for 16–18 minutes. Remove from the oven and put aside. The salmon is equally excellent, hot, or cold in the salad. Cook the salmon skin-side down and remove the salmon from the skin

using a fish slice after cooking. It should slide off easily when cooked.

- In a bowl, mix the mayonnaise, yogurt, rice wine vinegar, mint leaves, salt, and pepper and let it rest for at least 5 minutes, so the flavors develop.

- Arrange the salad leaves and spinach on a serving plate, then top with radishes, cucumber, onions, and parsley. Next, flake the cooked salmon onto the salad and drizzle the dressing over.

52. FRAGRANT ASIAN HOTPOT

Ingredients:

- 1 tsp tomato purée
- 1 crushed star anise or 1/4 tsp ground anise
- a small handful (10g) parsley, finely chopped

- a small handful (10g) coriander, finely chopped
- the juice of 1/2 lime
- 500 ml of fresh chicken stock
- 1/2 peeled carrot, cut into matchsticks
- 50g broccoli florets
- 50g beansprouts
- 100g raw tiger prawns
- 100g firm tofu, chopped
- 50g rice noodles, cooked according to instructions
- 50g cooked water chestnuts
- 20g chopped sushi ginger
- 1 tbsp miso paste

Instructions:

- Put the tomato purée, star anise, parsley, coriander, lime juice, and chicken stock in a pan, then bring to a simmer for about 10 minutes.

• Add the carrot, broccoli, prawns, tofu, noodles, and water chestnuts and simmer gently until the prawns are cooked through. Next, remove from the heat, then stir in the ginger and miso paste.

• Serve sprinkled with the parsley and coriander leaves.

53. LAMB, BUTTERNUT SQUASH AND DATE TAGINE

The incredible Moroccan spices will make this healthy tagine perfect for chilly autumn and winter evenings. To be served with buckwheat for an extra health kick!

Ingredients:

- 2 tablespoons of olive oil
- 1 sliced red onion
- 2cm of grated ginger
- 3 grated garlic cloves
- 1 teaspoon chili flakes
- 2 teaspoons of cumin seeds
- 1 cinnamon stick
- 2 teaspoons of ground turmeric
- 800g lamb neck fillet, cut into chunks
- 1/2 teaspoon salt
- 100g chopped Medjool dates
- 400g tin chopped tomatoes, plus half a can of water
- 500g butternut squash, chopped into cubes
- 400g tin chickpeas
- 2 tablespoons fresh coriander (plus extra for garnish)

- buckwheat, couscous, flatbreads or rice for the serving

Instructions:

- Preheat your oven to 284°F.

- Next drizzle about 2 tablespoons of oil into an ovenproof saucepan or cast iron casserole dish. Add the sliced onion and cook on a gentle heat, for about 5 minutes or until the onions are softened.

- Now add the grated garlic, ginger, chili, cumin, cinnamon, and turmeric. Stir well and cook for another minute. You may add a splash of water if it gets too dry.

- Next, add in the lamb chunks, then stir well to coat the meat in the onions and then add salt, chopped dates, and tomatoes, plus about half a can of water (100-200ml).

- Bring the tagine to the boil and put it in your preheated oven for at least 1 hour.

- Thirty minutes before the end of the cooking time, add in the butternut squash and chickpeas. Stir everything together and return to the oven for another 30 minutes.

- When the tagine is ready, remove from the oven, then stir through the chopped coriander. To be served with buckwheat, couscous, flatbreads, or basmati rice.

54. GRAPE AND MELON JUICE

Ingredients:

- 1/2 cucumber, peeled, halved, and roughly chopped
- 30g young spinach leaves
- 100g red seedless grapes

- 100g cantaloupe melon, deseeded and cut into chunks

Instructions:

- Blend all the ingredients in a juicer or blender until smooth.

55. GRILLED BEEF WITH A RED WINE SAUCE, ONION RINGS, GARLIC, KALE, AND HERB ROASTED POTATOES

Ingredients:

- 100g potatoes, peeled and diced
- 1 tbsp of extra virgin olive oil
- 5g chopped parsley
- 50g red onion, sliced into rings
- 50g kale, sliced
- 1 chopped garlic clove

- 120–150g x 3.5cm-thick beef fillet steak or sirloin steak

- 40ml of red wine

- 150ml beef stock

- 1 tsp tomato purée

- 1 tsp cornflour, dissolved in 1 tbsp water

Instructions:

- Heat the oven to 428ºF.

- Place the potatoes in a saucepan of boiling water, cook for 4–5 minutes, then drain. Place them in a roasting tin with 1 teaspoon of the oil and roast in the hot oven for about 35–45 minutes. Turn the potatoes every 10 minutes for even cooking. When the potatoes are cooked, remove from the oven, then sprinkle with the parsley and mix well.

- Now, fry the onion in 1 teaspoon of the oil over medium heat for 5–7 minutes or until soft and nicely caramelized. Keep it warm. Next, steam the kale for 2–3 minutes, then drain. Gently fry the garlic in ½ teaspoon of oil for 1 minute, until soft. Now, add the kale and cook for another 1–2 minutes, just until tender. Keep warm.

- Next, heat an ovenproof frying pan over high heat just until smoking. Coat the meat in ½ a teaspoon of oil, then fry in the hot pan over medium-high heat according to how you like it done.

- Remove the meat from the pan and put it aside to rest. Now, add the wine to the hot pan to bring up any meat residue. Let it bubble to reduce the wine by half, until syrupy.

- Finally, add the stock and tomato purée to the pan, bring to the boil, then add the cornflour paste to thicken your sauce, adding it a little at a time until you have your desired consistency. Stir in any of the juices from the steak, then serve with the roasted potatoes, kale, onion rings, and red wine sauce.

Simple exercises to maximize weight loss

When you follow a diet, no matter what type, you must combine it with physical activity. The Sirtfood Diet does not require exhausting gym exercises.

The physical exercise controls the changes in the cellular antioxidant system, mitochondrial biogenesis, and oxidative metabolism.

The skeletal muscles are involved both in movement and in endocrine activities. It means that they control the function of other organs, by their ability to secrete cytokines and transcription factors into the bloodstream.

The skeletal muscles contain 40% of the body weight, which means that insulin-stimulated uptake of glucose and the main energy-consuming lipid catabolism take place in the skeletal muscles.

The metabolic flexibility is essential to preserve metabolic homeostasis and other physiological processes, by merely switching glucose into lipid oxidation.

Sirtuins are affected by the cellular metabolic stress that comes from physical exercise. So, they have a vital role in controlling every cellular activity.

Therefore, activating sirtuins through physical exercise will enhance biogenesis and mitochondrial oxidative capacity, which is the essential factor in weight loss and overall well-being.

Except for calorie restriction, there are a few methods, simple ones, to maintain your body active throughout the entire process. And these are:

1. Walking

It is the most efficient and easy way for beginners to start exercising without feeling overwhelmed. It is estimated that 165 calories are burned per 30 minutes of walking at a moderate pace. In small words, walking for 50-70 minutes 3 times a week reduces body fat by an average of 1.5%.

To get started, try to add more steps to your day, take the stairs at work, or to take your dog for extra walks for at least 30 minutes a day.

You will gradually increase the frequency of your walk as you go further with your diet.

2. Jogging or running

These exercises are bound to make you lose weight. The difference between them is that a jogging pace is between 4-6 miles/h, while running is faster than 6 miles/h.

It is estimated that 298 calories are burned per 30 minutes of jogging and 372 per 30 minutes of running.

Furthermore, running and jogging helps us burn belly fat, which is linked to chronic diseases like diabetes and heart disease.

To get started, aim to jog for 20-30 minutes a day, 3-4 times a week. In time you will increase the duration and frequency of your jogging or running sessions.

3. Cycling

Traditionally cycling is done outdoors, but many gyms and fitness centers have stationary bikes for indoor exercise. Thank God for that! We can cycle while storm or rain runs through the town!

It is estimated that 260 calories are burned per 30 minutes cycling on a stationary bike or 298 calories per 30 minutes on a bicycle at a moderate pace(13.9 miles/hour).

Studies have shown that regular cycling leads to overall fitness, increased insulin sensitivity, and lower risk of cancer, heart disease, and death.

4. Weight training

Weight training is very sought after by those who want to build strength and promote muscle growth.

It is estimated that 112 calories per 30 minutes are burned during weight training.

It also helps us increase the metabolic rate (RMR)- in small words, how many calories your body burns at rest.

Studies have found that 125 additional calories are burned per day and that our bodies burn calories many hours after a weight-training workout.

5. Interval training

Interval training, also known as high-intensity interval training (HIIT), refers to short bursts of intense exercise that alternate with recovery periods.

Usually, it takes 30 seconds of intense exercise and rest times.

Studies have shown that HIIT helps us burn 25-30% more calories per minute than cycling, running, or weight training exercises.

The good news is that HIIT is easy to incorporate in our daily exercise routine. All you have to do is choose a type of exercise and the rest times. For example, try to run as fast as you can fr 30 seconds, then slow down for 1-2 minutes. Repeat for 10-30 minutes in a row.

6. Swimming

Swimming is one of the complete sports, just like tennis. You get to engage a vast area of muscles while doing it.

It is estimated that 233 calories are burned in 30 minutes of swimming.

Studies have shown that 60 minutes 3 times a week of swimming leads to significant weight loss, decreased heart disease risk, and improved flexibility.

7. Yoga

Yoga is a popular way to relieve stress. It helps us burn a fair amount of calories and offers additional health benefits.

It is estimated that 149 calories are burned per 30 minutes of practicing yoga.

A 12-week study has shown that two 90-minute yoga sessions a week led to waist circumference reduction by an average of 1.5 inches.

Furthermore, subjects have experienced improvements in mental and physical well-being, such as overeating control, mindfulness eating, and understanding the body's hunger signals.

The good news is that you can also practice yoga at home with guided tutorials.

8. Pilates

Pilates makes you burn 108 calories in a 30-minute session.

Studies have shown that in 8 weeks, performing Pilates exercises for 90 minutes, 3 times a week leads to a significantly reduced waist, lower back pain, improved strength, flexibility, and endurance.

The good news is that you can practice Pilates at home, any time, with no harmful effects on your overall well-being.

All these exercises have different results for everyone. There are no two people alike.

Besides that, we must consider other aspects. They are:

- Age. Older people tend to carry less muscle mass. That leads to reduced RMR, so, losing weight becomes more difficult.

- Genetics. Some people are prone to weigh more. Genes are tricky. No matter the efforts, some tend to shed more pounds than others. Rapid weight loss can lead to dehydration, headaches, irritability, and fatigue.

- Gender. Men tend to lose more weight than women, and most certainly, in less time.

- Sleep. Lack of sleep slows the rate of weight loss and increases the cravings for unhealthy foods.

- Medical conditions. Unfortunately, people with depression or hypothyroidism have to put up with extra efforts to lose weight.

Conclusions

The Sirtfood Diet seems like a miracle for those who want to lose weight fast. We have seen that it works and why it works!

We have learned about the power of sirtuins, the ability of antique food cultures and lifestyles that in our days seem so unreachable. Even if we live in modern times, always in a hurry, always in search of some elixir of endless youth, the best thing to do is take a look at our ancestors and how they simply enjoyed life, with the simplest things, foods, and concerns about the future.

We have also seen the cons and pros. The star testimonials are maybe those that make us try almost anything in life! Following our idols' lifestyle sounds better for each one of us!

The truth is people have always undergone strange, most restrictive diets (and lots of them!) for a false idea of living a "happily ever after" life with great body shape- the iconic body shape, let's say!

Well, the first thing to do is to realize that each one of us is unique. No diet, no physical exercise will ever have the same results for two different people. Never!

We can try this innovative method since it's quite harmless- except for the calorie restriction. But, with the guidance of a dietitian or general practitioner, we have nothing to worry. We all know how much we are thriving for acceptance and public approval. So, let's give it a try! Maybe it is the perfect solution for you!

Since you get to eat plenty of delicious foods, chocolate and drink red wine, maybe you should consider it! Let's get French!

Do Not Go Yet! One Last Thing To Do!
If you enjoyed this book or found it useful, I'd be very grateful if you'd post a short review on Amazon. Your support does make a difference, and I read all the reviews personally so I can get your feedback and make this book even better.

Thanks for your help and support!